PRACTICAL HYDROTHERAPY

A Home Guide to Water Cure Treatment

by

Gerhard Leibold

Translated from the German by Transcript

THORSONS PUBLISHERS LIMITED
Wellingborough, Northamptonshire

First published in Germany as
gesund und fit durch die Kneippkur zu Hause
© Walter Hädecke Verlag, Weil der Stadt 1979
First published in English in 1980

British Library Cataloguing in Publication Data

Leibold, Gerhard
   Practical hydrotherapy.
   1. Hydrotherapy
   I. Title
   615'.853   RM811

   ISBN 0-7225-0656-2

Photoset by Promenade Graphics Ltd., Cheltenham,
Gloucestershire.
Printed and bound in Great Britain by
Weatherby Woolnough, Wellingborough, Northamptonshire.

CONTENTS

		Page
Foreword	... ...	7

Chapter

Part One: THE KNEIPP VIEW OF HEALTHY LIVING

1.	Total Treatment	9

Part Two: BASIC PRINCIPLES

2.	Home Treatment	14
3.	Compresses and Packs	22
4.	Affusions	35
5.	Jets	43
6.	Baths	46
7.	Vapour Treatments	52
8.	Gymnastics and Sport	60
9.	Air and Sun Baths	64
10.	A Well-balanced Diet	66

Part Three: MEDICAL INDICATIONS

11.	Vegetative and Mental Disorders	72
12.	Disorders of the Heart, Circulation and Blood Vessels	77
13.	Digestive and Metabolic Disturbances ...	82
14.	Diseases of the Bones and Joints and other Disorders	87
15.	Home Aids to Health	92
	Index	96

FOREWORD

This book is not intended to be a professional instruction manual. It is designed for those who would like to use the healing forces of nature in their own homes, in order to strengthen the body's vitality and aid its restorative powers. Here, Kneipp's system of health and healing is outlined in simple terms to make it readily accessible to the general reader.

The book is also meant for those who have been taking the Kneipp Cure and would like to continue the treatment themselves. Not everything that is done at the hydro is suitable for the ordinary household. At home there is usually neither the time nor the necessary expert supervision available. Therefore, discussion has been confined to those measures which anyone can carry out without difficulty or danger, including, most emphatically, adopting a well-balanced diet and taking plenty of exercise in the open air.

The Kneipp water treatments appropriate for the home are those which are not too demanding and those that do not require special apparatus; in other words, such treatments as arm and foot baths, partial affusions to knee or shoulder level, compresses on the arms, legs, chest, shins and calves, body compresses and packs, not forgetting the use of such items as the 'mashed-potato bag'.

Douches and water-treading are also recommended for domestic use. Finally, time-honoured herbal remedies are advocated in place of tablets for colds, the odd bout of insomnia and simple stomach upsets, when these have no serious impact on the general health.

The Reverend Kneipp earned himself the nickname of 'the watering-can parson of Wörishofen' because of his water treatments. All the same, he was not the inventor of water therapy. The healing power of water was well known before the time of Christ, but Kneipp established hydrotherapy as a means of cure adaptable to each disease and each type of constitution and this sets him apart from his predecessors.

In contrast to many other lay practitioners, he did not regard his own speciality (in this case water) as a cure-all. He was always urging his contemporaries to return to a coarse, well-balanced, nutritious diet—advice which is even more pertinent today. Other basic features of his teachings were gymnastics and sport—carefully adapted to the physical strength of the individual—air and sun baths and herbal remedies, nearly all of which he proved on himself before recommending them to his patients. As a minister of religion, Kneipp did not forget the importance of spiritual health in relation to the health of the body, and in this course he has been vindicated by the findings of modern psychosomatic medicine.

Thus the Kneipp system consists of health care and healing by the joint action of water, exercise, light, air, diet and herbs. Thus, it is never restricted to treating one symptom or one part of the body. It is whole man who suffers and the whole man who needs to be treated. Even in applications to individual parts of the body, this principle is observed, because there is a reaction from the part treated on the body as a whole.

Many patients, year after year, derive renewed vitality from the Kneipp Cure. The suggestions in this book can help them to consolidate the results and prevent a relapse. And those who have no chance of taking the cure will find here a health programme for improving or regaining their health without great expense. Our hope is that this book will aid the seeker to become an active whole in the sense understood by Kneipp.

GERHARD LEIBOLD
Institute for Psychology and Natural Healing,
Karlsruhe.

PART ONE

THE KNEIPP VIEW OF HEALTHY LIVING

CHAPTER 1

TOTAL TREATMENT

As far as most people are concerned, the Kneipp Cure is the same as a cold water cure, and they hardly know anything of his other thinking. It is quite true that the use of water was prominent in his healing system, but in addition he gave advice on sensible feeding and living, without which his cure was incomplete. The Kneipp Cure is a total treatment, for not only is therapy applied locally to the diseased part of the body but there is an indeterminate spreading of the effect throughout the whole organism. The self-healing mechanism of the body is activated. This means that the illness is not overcome passively by the application of drugs, but actively by the organism itself. It is quite obvious that, with this improved defence, not only can acute disorders be healed but new diseases can be circumvented—a very welcome advantage.

Holistic Therapy
Kneipp treatments, since they act on the body as a whole, cannot be successfully applied to certain disorders. Generally speaking, the treatments are no substitute for surgery and there are several diseases which require specific therapies. But, even so, it can be confidently

9

maintained that the body that has been strengthened by Kneipp applications will fare better than one which has been pampered.

The Rev. Kneipp was no crotchety eccentric, as is sometimes found amongst unorthodox practitioners. He did not insist that the procedure he had developed was the sole method of effective therapy. And he was certainly not the charlatan or quack doctor, that many orthodox doctors of his day claimed him to be; rather he endeavoured from quite early on to familiarize the medical profession with his methods so that they might benefit from his own experience and then develop it further in the light of new knowledge. Kneipp was and remained a pastor first and foremost and came into daily contact with human failings. Also, he was too conscious of his own weaknesses as an ordinary human being to expect too much of his patients. His methods of healing are not one-sided and they do not require excessive self-discipline on the part of the patients. Perhaps this is one reason why his methods have been so popular?

Kneipp saw amazing medical advances made in his lifetime. For the very first time, bacteria had been unmasked as the causes of many diseases. Over-reacting to this success, people were inclined to forget that the patient is a whole entity and to treat him as a kind of machine with faulty parts. Under the influence of this blind obsession, medical men overlooked the fact that not everyone with a complaint is suffering from some infection and also that the individual predisposition to disease which, in part, is due to the psyche and, in part, to wrong feeding and mode of life, has a role to play too. It was at this time, moreover, that many valuable herbs began to be neglected.

The Rev. Kneipp, with his practical, matter-of-fact approach, ran counter to this trend towards specialization found in the allopathic doctors. He had a well-known saying to the effect that 'the good host throws out unwanted guests himself'! In other words, when the organism is strengthened, the sufferer can overcome the disease by using his own resources. Only now are ordinary medical men beginning, somewhat reluctantly, to return to the idea of treating the whole man. No doubt a certain amount of credit is due to Kneipp's teachings for this.

Hydrotherapy

The renown of Rev. Kneipp is based mainly on his expertise with the 'watering can' as folk thought of it, even though this was only one part of his life's work. He came to hydrotherapy through his own illness. He was suffering from tuberculosis and the doctor had already given him up for dead. In spite of this gloomy prognosis, he was completely cured by the healing action of water. And the way in which he tried to pass on the benefits of his own experience to others, shows the far-sightedness of this medical layman who had no formal training. Although his own experience might well have prompted him to regard water as a 'cure-all', he did not stop there. He realized that because the rather drastic course of treatment he had taken had worked for him, this did not mean that it was generally applicable to all other sufferers and diseases. Thus, he refined the water cure by many new methods, most of which he discovered himself, until it became the individually adaptable form of treatment we know today.

Prevention is Better than Cure

However, Kneipp's doctrine of health is not restricted to healing the sick. He had something of the spirit of the old Asiatic physicians, who were paid only so long as the patients remained fit and well—a state of affairs demanding considerably more care than that provided by our modern medical practitioners. Kneipp was a great believer in the saying, 'prevention is better than cure'. This was a leading thought in all his methods. His idea was to support or renew the 'vital force' of the human organism in such a way that the body could fight the disease in its own strength. Stimulation with water is only one possibility here. Kneipp regarded *natural living* and *correct feeding* as at least equally important.

Feeding

Basically, correct feeding is quite easy. All that is required is to eat a varied diet of raw or carefully prepared food that is as simple as possible. Refined foodstuffs, excessive meat-eating and any other one-sidedness in the diet are to be avoided as far as possible. This coarse, mixed diet has become even more important today because, in spite of food surpluses, more and more people are complaining of deficiencies in their nutrition. Kneipp's intuitions are becoming increasingly confirmed by present-day dieticians. A proper regime means, above all, a right attitude to life. Open-air exercise, sun and air baths and hardening the body with applications of water are not sufficient safeguards. It is true that these are valuable measures but they are incomplete without a reformed attitude to life and to our fellow-men.

Attitude to Life
It is necessary today, more than ever in the history of mankind, to get back into harmony with our surroundings, to abandon our strife against animate and inanimate nature, to cease looking upon others as competitors at our place of work or possible rivals in private life. What we need is to have respect and human warmth for our fellows and a proper regard for nature. Symptomatic of our false attitudes are the impending energy and raw materials crises, the increasing sense of alienation afflicting modern man and the vague fears that plague and cripple him.

Kneipp's advocacy of moderation, simplicity and temperance in all areas of life are yet another indication of his far-sightedness and of his realization that it is not enough to heal the body but that the mind needs treatment too, if health is to be recovered permanently. Once again, the pastor in Kneipp comes to the fore, knowing as he did that we are daily exposed to diseases which will make us irrevocably ill and disturbed, if we do not approach one another with new attitudes and expectations.

Whoever is content to treat man materialistically as a highly complicated machine with various faulty parts, will, even with the best of drugs and the most modern of apparatus, do no more than alleviate the suffering for a time without achieving true healing. The plethora of psy-

chosomatic diseases presented by those who frequent
our doctors' waiting rooms — that is to say, troubles of
the body originating in the mind — are becoming
increasingly common and prove how topical Kneipp's
doctrine of health still remains.

Now this does not mean that the Kneipp Cure is fit only
for such psychosomatic diseases, even though it often
achieves amazing results with these stubborn troubles. A
favourable effect is obtained with the Kneipp treatments
in practically all illnesses where an operation or radiation
therapy is not indicated; at the very least the action of
other remedies is actively promoted. Among those which
might be mentioned as the diseases that can be helped
include those of the heart, blood vessels, circulation,
general metabolism, digestive system, skin, muscles and
bones.

PART TWO

BASIC PRINCIPLES

CHAPTER 2

HOME TREATMENT

This book is intended for those who would like to carry out the Kneipp treatment at home in order to prevent or treat various illnesses, and for those who wish to live more rationally and naturally. It is also suitable for the reader who has already experienced the benefits of the cure at a Kneipp hydro and does not wish to lose them.

This book is certainly not an adviser on self-treatment without medical examination and advice. Because there are so many possible forms of application, the correct choice and conduct of the treatment are of critical importance. This choice should be left to an experienced practitioner. So when we speak of home treatment, we do not mean treatment unaided, with no proper guidance. Of course, there is nothing to be said against occasional recourse to the 'wet sock' treatment for insomnia, or the use of a cold arm bath as a refresher on a hot day, without seeking the doctor's advice. Curative treatments, however, are quiet another matter and require a definite plan of campaign worked out and controlled by the physician.

The function of this book is to instruct the reader so that he can correctly carry out what the doctor orders; for even the best plan of treatment is worth little when the techniques required to put it into practice have not been properly mastered. Any directions that are not clearly understood, especially when they concern important procedures, should be left to the trained spa attendant. At home, only the simpler methods should be attempted, and these too must be employed properly.

No Excesses
Everywhere we look we see people who tend to carry things to excess. In the first place they lead lives that fly in the face of common sense, and then they try to counteract the consequences of their behaviour by taking an excess of health precautions. Witness the increasing abuse of medicinal tablets. And what goes for tablets, goes for the Kneipp Cure. The saying, 'the more the better' is always wrong. An organism that has forgotten how to react properly to natural stimuli, will most definitely be overloaded when treated with strong measures or by several applications at the same time. There is surely no need to stress the point that time is needed. What has taken years to go wrong, cannot be put right in a few days. According to the 'basic biological law' of the psychologist, Arndt, and the pharmacologist, Schulz, the weak stimuli assist us much more, while overstrong stimuli, to which we are unaccustomed, inhibit us and do us harm. Therefore, in domestic use, the Kneipp Cure starts with mild local applications. The individual reaction to these is observed and discussed with the practitioner. He alone will be able to judge whether and when more vigorous means are indicated.

The Healing Crisis
The healing crisis is one possible reaction in the course of the treatment. It is to be seen most of all in obstinate, chronic diseases. This crisis signals, with an aggravation of the discomfort, that the body's defences have been brought to their peak of activity and that healing will follow. This is the only way in which many diseases may be overcome. So when there is a temporary aggravation of the trouble during the course of treatment, this is an

indication to call in the doctor, not to discontinue the treatment as a failure. In this way he can make an assessment and decide on a further therapy, with a view to promoting rather than suppressing the crisis, so that the healing will be total.

The object of the cure is to influence the mental attitude as well as the body. This is hard to do as long as one fails to detach oneself from everyday problems. Anyone who has undergone autogenic training or knows some relaxation technique of any sort, certainly has an advantage here. If possible the course of treatment should be commenced during a holiday and then the applications can be continued in the working week.

Water Applications: A Brief History
Water was already held in high repute as a healing agent by the physician priests of Ancient Egypt, and the Persians used curative baths. Ancient Rome, too, was famous for its highly cultivated use of baths. With the fall of the Roman Empire, the application of water as a remedy was gradually forgotten. In the 'water-shy' Europe of the Middle Ages, washing oneself with water was actually considered vulgar by the nobility.

It was not until the eighteenth century that Dr Sigmund Hahn of Schweidnitz and his son, Johann Sigmund Hahn, rediscovered the curative power of water. They were popularly known in Germany as the *Wasser-Hähne* or water taps in punning reference to their surname, *Hahn*, a tap; however they were not able to make hydrotherapy a recognized part of orthodox medicine.

This honour also eluded the farmer's son Vincenz Priessnitz, who took the therapy still further. This eccentric individual, who was described as taciturn, morose and uncouth by his contemporaries, placed too much emphasis on cold water and coarse food. What is more, he failed to see that his spartan treatment was not suitable for every disease or every patient. Priessnitz used to take a close and critical look at those who wished to be admitted to the hydro at his father's smallholding in Gräfenberg and is said often to have refused treatment without reference to the condition or appearance of his patients. In spite of his indisputable success, he was unable to gain official recognition for his treatment.

It was not until the arrival of the Rev. Sebastian Kneipp on the scene that water therapy really came to the fore again. Kneipp first saw the light of day in the year 1821 in Stefansried. He started out to become a weaver but soon felt he had a vocation for the priesthood and began to study for it. When he fell ill with tuberculosis of the lungs, the doctors quickly decided that his case was hopeless, but the 'candidate for death' as he called himself, did not give up easily. The writings of the Hahns were placed in his hands and he began to treat himself. Presumably, he was indebted to a constitution that was still robust, in spite of his consumption, for surviving the *rigors* of dips in the ice-cold waters of the Donau without permanent injury to his health. In fact he made a complete recovery notwithstanding the doctors' prognoses. This experience was the basis of his work, which was to make him world-famous. With great resolution, Kneipp tested the various ways of applying water and numerous herbal remedies on himself and so eventually worked out his method of treatment, with which nearly all diseases could be favourably influenced. What is more, in his book, *How You Should Live*, he showed how to prevent many of those health problems which are nowadays known as diseases of civilization.

In contrast to many other medical outsiders, Kneipp avoided any kind of one-sidedness. Therefore he did not refuse to consider the use of warm water and was not one-sided in his approach to matters of diet and many other questions. One of his most notable services was the introduction of affusions to hydrotherapy. This earned him the nickname of 'the watering-can parson'. Parson Kneipp developed, out of the simple applications of water of the Hahns and the rather unbalanced treatments of Priessnitz, a sophisticated therapy which was adaptable to any constitution and any individual disease. This was the first time that it became possible to determine the exact amounts of water required in each case, as had long been done with other remedies.

Strictly speaking, it is not from the water itself that we

should expect to obtain benefit, although possibly its stimulus may prove helpful in certain diseases. No, in the Kneipp applications, the most important factor is the temperature of the water. When there is hardly any difference between water and body temperature, that is to say when the temperature of the water lies between 35°C/95°F and 37°C/99°F, scarcely any effect can be found. Hence baths at these temperatures are fit only for washing in. Water temperature and pressure evoke a reaction from the blood vessels, nerves and metabolic functions. At least one of these systems is affected in almost every disease. That is why hydrotherapy can favourably influence virtually every disease although, of course, it is better for some things than for others.

Warm and Cold Water Treatment
Hot water at temperatures of more than 37°C/99°F is indicated when the patient is too unreactive or infirm for cold applications, and especially when the body temperature is below normal. The blood vessels relax under the influence of the heat, the blood pressure falls and the individual feels tired and at ease. Hot applications should always be followed by a cold shower or wash.

Cold water works through the *reaction of the body* to the stimulation of the cold, not through the coldness itself as is often thought. This stimulation raises the blood pressure, the blood supply is improved, the whole metabolism is activated and the nervous system is animated. The part of the body treated experiences a comforting glow and the skin itself often reddens. Cold applications should not be carried out except on a well-warmed body and in an adequately heated room. Should the patient feel chilly or unwell at any stage, the application must be immediately discontinued, and he must be quickly warmed up either by exercise or by tucking him up in bed. The duration of cold applications is governed by the onset of the reaction, that is to say, by a reddening of the skin or by the short sharp pang of cold that is followed by a sensation of warmth.

At the end of a water application one usually dries only the hair and the places between the toes (because of the risk of foot fungus). The water is just wiped from the rest of the body with the hand, after which, one either 'steams off' in bed for a short while, or dresses and warms up and dries out under ones clothes fairly quickly while doing some exercises. Only in exceptional cases may the body be dried straight away.

Although hydrotherapy is often used to treat selected parts of the body only, it is nevertheless a total therapy. The whole organism is influenced via its parts. Many of the applications are each specially indicated in certain complaints, but there are no cut-and-dried formulas of affusions, baths and so on for every disease. The particular form a treatment will take always depends on the general condition and reaction of the patient.

Healing takes place through stimulation of the metabolic processes, the nervous system and the circulation. In this way, the whole body is strengthened, its defences are mobilized and its self-healing tendency assisted.

Rubbing

For rubbing, one requires a cold, wet sheet that has been well wrung out. The sheet should be fairly thick. The whole body or that part of the body which is being treated should be enveloped in this sheet without puckering the latter if possible. It must cling tight and smooth to the surface of the skin, ready for rubbing strongly with both hands. The stimulus of the cold and the mechanical rubbing are both effective in their own way.

The order of procedure is as follows: back of right hand, back of arm upwards to the shoulder, arm and chest front and back; the left-hand side in the same way. For a complete rub, follow with right foot, outside and inside of leg, sole of foot; the left-hand side in the same way. Finally the buttocks and trunk are rubbed down.

After the rubbing is over, the patient is dried vigorously with a turkish towel and tucked up in a warm bed for a half to one hour. Four to six treatments can be given daily, or more frequently if the doctor approves.

Rub-downs are gently strengthening and stimulate the circulation and the metabolism.

Washing
In washing, the part of the body being treated is not wrapped in a wet sheet, but is washed with a really damp, but not dripping, coarse linen cloth.

When washing the upper body, the order of procedure

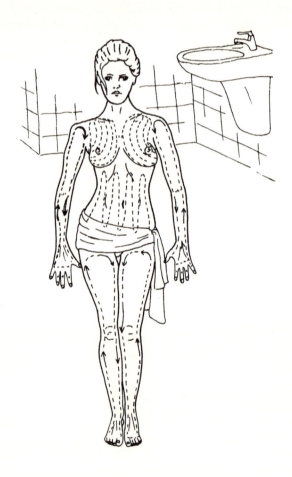

Fig. 1. Rubbing and Washing

is as follows: back of right hand, outside and inside of arm; left side as right. The chest and back are washed next. The cloth is dipped and wrung out again four times in all.

In washing the lower body, start on the right in this order: foot, outside leg to hip and back down on inside, back of leg, sole of foot, cover leg. The left-hand side is treated in the same way.

In washing the whole body the washing of the upper body is combined with that of the lower body.

With bedridden patients one part of the body is kept covered while the other part is being washed. In lower-body and whole-body washing the cloth is wet and wrung out again six times in all.

When the washing is over, the patient goes to bed for half an hour or an hour or warms and dries his freshly clothed body as quickly as possible by moving about.

Experience has shown that washing in this way is good for hardening the body without overstraining it, for reducing fevers, for nervous debility and nervous excitement, for insomnia and circulatory disturbances. In fevers, the applications should be made every one or two hours, otherwise up to four times a day. Even feeble adults and children respond well to the washing without coming to any harm.

The action of the rubbing and washing can be strengthened by using vinegar-water (1 part vinegar to three parts water).

CHAPTER 3

COMPRESSES AND PACKS

Three cloths are always needed for compresses and packs: the wet cloth of coarse linen which is laid directly on the skin, a somewhat larger linen cloth that is laid over that, and a still larger woollen blanket on the outside. Practitioners have cloths cut to size for every type of use, but the ordinary householder will find linen cloths in the following sizes quite adequate:

190 × 210cm (6 × 7ft) for full compresses, chest-to-toe compresses.

160 × 180cm (5 × 6ft) for short compresses.

150 × 150cm (5 × 5ft) for the shawl.

80 × 180cm (2½ × 6ft) for packs, chest compresses, cross-over compresses, and loin compresses.

80 × 80cm (2½ × 2½ft) for foot compresses, shin compresses, calf compresses and head compresses.

60 × 90cm (2 × 3ft) for arm compresses.

60 × 60cm (2 × 2ft) for hand compresses.

20 × 60cm (8 × 24ins) for neck compresses.

No Puckers
In packs, the sheet is folded one or more times according to the region being treated and is applied to the body in such a way as to fit snugly without wrinkling. The dry

middle sheet and the woollen blanket are then placed on top.

In compresses too, any irritating wrinkles are carefully avoided in the wet sheet before the two dry covers are put on.

Compresses and packs are employed either with plain water or with water with additives.

In cold applications, vinegar (1 part to 3 of water), clay, salt—50g to 1 litre (1oz to 1 pint) of water— or curds are suitable additives. Herbal additives are used with hot packs and compresses.

The reaction will occur in one to two hours in the form of a perspiration and a pleasant warmth through whole or part of the body. If the object of the compress is to reduce a fever, it must be changed in good time before the patient gets too hot. As soon as the reaction has set in, the cloths are to be taken off, but the patient should remain in bed for another half an hour while he perspires gently. After this, he will have a cold shower or cold wash-down. If the patient starts to feel unwell during the application or begins to shiver, which would be more likely to happen with the big compresses (the full or chest-to-toe compresses), he must be rubbed dry immediately and be put to bed with hot water bottles or an electric blanket.

Cold Compresses
Cold packs and compresses stimulate the circulation, activate the metabolism, calm the nerves, alleviate sleep disorders and reduce fevers. Medical practitioners some-times use them to act on internal organs via the skin reflex zones.

Hot Compresses
Hot packs and compresses, the effect of which can be increased by the use of hot water bottles, relieve cramps and colics and soothe aches and pains.

Waterproof Sheets
Beginners with water treatments may find it advisable to spread a plastic sheet over the patient's mattress before proceeding. It would not be good for him to have to

sleep on a damp mattress and contract a chill or rheumatism after being relieved from some other trouble.

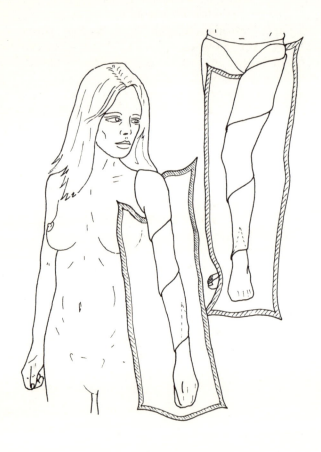

Fig. 2. Arm and Leg Compresses

Arm and Hand Compresses

The hand compresses encase the hand as far as the wrist. A square cloth is folded into a triangle and the middle corner is laid pointing forward on the back of the hand and the two remaining corners are firmly wound round the hand and wrist. The compress must fit firmly without constricting the hand or interfering with the circulation (*this is essential*).

In arm compresses, the arm and hand are enveloped in the wet sheet right up to the shoulder. The cloths are tucked in at the top of the arm in such a way that the longer end is on the outside and falls over the shoulder, while the shorter end finishes under the arm-pit.

Foot, Calf and Lower-leg Compresses

The foot compress is the same in principle as the hand compress. The square cloths are folded once to form triangles, the middle corner covers the back of the foot and the toes, the two outer corners are wrapped round the foot and ankle. Here too, the extremity is firmly covered without constricting it in any way.

Calf compresses, chiefly valued for reducing fevers, reach from the ankle to the knee-hollow. The foot itself is left free. In lower-leg compresses the calf compress is combined with the foot compress. However, in this case, the cloths are not folded into the triangle shape. After the foot has been wrapped as for the foot compress, the remainder of the cloth is used as for the calf compress in order to wrap the lower leg up to the knee-hollow.

Whole Leg Compresses

The whole-leg compress is the same as a lower-leg compress except that it is carried over the knee and as far as the hip. As in the arm compresses, the cloths must be splayed at the top so that the shorter side ends at the groin and the longer side folds over the hip.

Head Compresses

The head compress begins above the eyebrows and is wrapped around the skull apart from the neck. For this purpose, square cloths are folded into triangles. The central corner is laid back over the head and the two side corners cross one another at the back of the head and are tucked in at the front. Instead of using a wet cloth, the hair may be wetted and then covered with the dry linen cloth and woollen cloth. When the treatment is over the hair must be carefully dried.

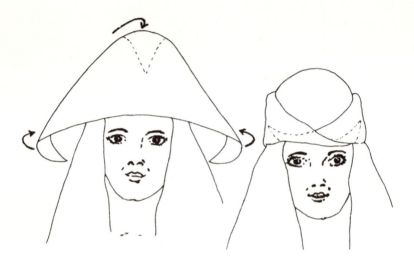

Fig. 3. Head Compresses

Neck Compresses
Neck compresses are made up of cloths folded once lengthwise and turned twice round the neck. When the symptoms are acute, the compress should be changed frequently, whereas in chronic diseases it may even be worn overnight.

Chest Compresses
The chest compress extends from the arm-pits to the costal arch. The three cloths are placed on the bed in such a way that the patient can lie down on the wet upper one. The patient is then carefully wrapped in them, care being taken not to restrict the breathing in any way.

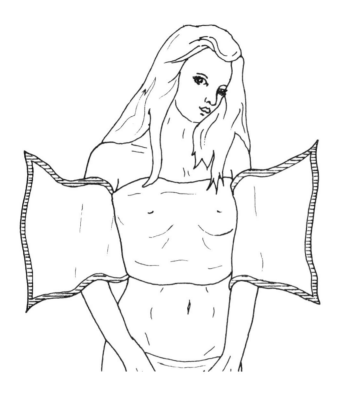

Fig. 4. Chest Compresses

Cross-over Compresses

For the cross-over compress one uses either a sufficiently long winding cloth that can be pulled out from the chest about 80cm (2½ft) on each side, or one takes three shorter cloths which can be wrapped round the chest and shoulders in a similar manner. The right-hand part of the wet cloth is passed under the right arm and over the left shoulder so as to cover the breast, and the left-hand part is similarly arranged. As will readily be seen, the two halves cross one another over the back (hence the name).

The dry linen cloth and the woollen blanket are used to cover the shoulders, upper arm and chest completely.

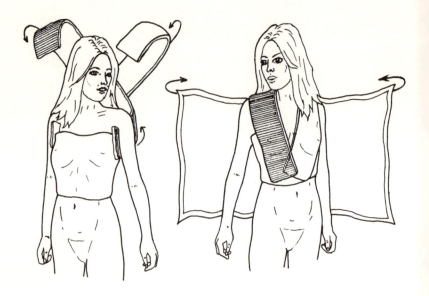

Fig. 5. Cross-over Compresses

Short Compress
The short compress reaches from the arm-pit to the knee-hollow. The cloths are arranged on the bed as described for the chest compress. The patient lies down on the wet sheet, which is of course on top, and is carefully enveloped in the wrappings.

Loin Compresses
Loin compresses differ from short compresses in that they reach only from the costal arch to the middle of the upper thigh.

Chest-to-toe Compresses
Chest-to-toe compresses envelop the body from the arm-pits to the feet, while the arms remain free. The wet cloth next to the skin is also pushed between the legs.

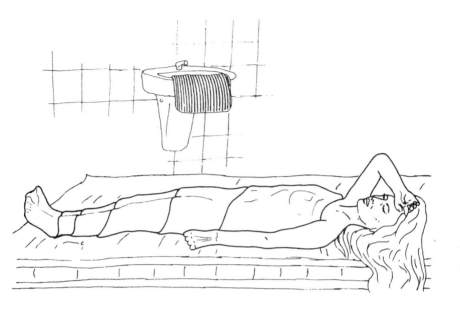

Fig. 6. Chest-to-toe Compresses

Full Compress

The full compress starts at the neck and reaches to the feet. It is difficult to apply and only an experienced nurse should attempt to do so. Full compresses, like chest-to-toe compresses, must always be applied in the morning and the condition of the patient must be kept under observation by an experienced assistant so that, if complications occur, the treatment can be discontinued at once and the appropriate countermeasures can be taken. Both these forms of compress must be avoided, unless one has the doctor's permission.

In full compresses a woollen blanket is first laid lengthwise on the bed and a second one is laid over it widthways. Over these comes the dry linen cloth and then the wet cloth used for swathing. At the upper end, the cloths are folded to a hands breadth for tucking in round the neck. After this preparation, the patient lies down on the cloths. His chest is covered with a wet cloth tucked in at the sides. Next, the neck and shoulders are enveloped in the large wet inside cloth, and after that the trunk and legs are too, to the tips of the toes. The dry cloth is wrapped on top in the same way. Finally, the woollen blanket lying crossways is used to cover the upper body and the other blanket is used to cover the legs.

For hot full compresses, the woollen blankets and dry cloth are first heated with hot water bottles, the inside cloth is dipped in hot water at 60°C/140°F and the patient is wrapped as described above. The head and face are covered with a wet cotton cloth, leaving only the nose and mouth free, and this cloth is covered in the same way by two woollen cloths. Finally the body is covered with a feather-bed or three woollen blankets. The damp cloth is removed briefly every half an hour in order to rewet it. After two hours the wrappings are removed, and the patient is left to perspire in a warm bed for another hour at least. Immediately afterwards he should put on pyjamas or a night-shirt, ready for a rest of several more hours. In dry full compresses, a dry inner cloth is used instead of the wet one.

The Shirt
In practice, the shirt resembles the full compress. Instead of a cloth, one uses for the inner, wet part of the compress a long linen shirt with long sleeves reaching down to the knuckles. This is wetted and the patient quickly puts it on and lies down on the dry cloths on his bed. The shirt is pushed in firmly between his legs so that it clings to the skin. The hands, feet and head are not covered. The dry cloths are applied as for the full compress.

The Spanish Cloak
The Spanish Cloak is another form of the full compress. Like the shirt, it is obtainable from specialist shops. It differs from the shirt in that it comes down over the feet and the tips of the fingers.

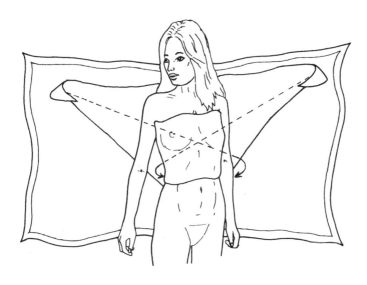

Fig. 7. The Shawl

The Shawl

The shawl is made from a large, square-cut linen cloth. This is folded to form a triangle. It is wetted and its long side is laid over the patient's neck and shoulders in such a way that the middle corner covers the back while the two remaining corners stick out on each side. The patient then lies down on the dry cloths which have been spread out on his bed. The nurse tugs on the two outside corners so that the shawl envelops the back firmly without puckering. The breast is covered with a damp cloth that is tucked in tight between the sides of the chest and the arms. One of the free corners of the shawl is next pulled across the arm and chest to the other side of the body, where it is tucked in between the arm and the trunk. The second free corner is then pulled over the front of the body to its opposite side and tucked in over the outside of the corresponding arm. The dry cloths are then wrapped round the outside, care being taken that there is a good seal at the neck without pulling them too tight.

Wet Socks

The Rev. Kneipp prized the wet sock treatment very highly. This is simpler to apply than the standard foot compress. Cotton socks replace the wet inner cloth and a pair of dry socks are pulled over these. The dry socks (or the usual dry linen cloth and woollen blanket) should cover the tops of the wet socks by several centimetres.

Compresses with Additives

Clay can be used either as a paste or as clay-water. Usually a finger-thick layer of cold clay paste is employed instead of the wet cloth. Over this come the dry cloth and the woollen blanket. An application lasts for one to two hours. As soon as the clay begins to crumble, the treatment is ended with a short cold washdown. The clay shirt is simply the shirt dipped in clay water and then put on as usual.

Salt shirts, which are particularly indicated in nervous debility, are dipped in a solution of 50g salt to 1 litre water (1 oz to 1 pint) and worn in the usual way.

Compresses with curds are prepared firstly by straining the curds through a sieve. The curds are whipped in water into a sort of salve and this paste is spread, finger-thick, on the compress cloth, which is applied as usual, followed by the two dry covers.

Body Packs

The pack consists of a cloth folded two to six times and applied, as wrinkle-free as possible, between the costal arch and the upper thighs. As in the compresses, a dry cloth and woollen blanket are laid on top. These packs have a particularly favourable influence on the organs of digestion.

Front Packs and Back Packs

Front packs cover the body from the arm-pits to the knees and back packs cover the back of the body from the shoulders to the knee-hollows. The dry cloth and the

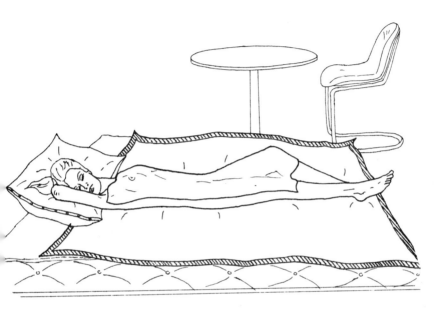

Fig. 8. Packs

outer woollen blanket are placed on top just as in the compresses.

Back packs are suitable for diseases of the spinal column and spinal cord, for lung affections, nervous debility. Front packs are good for lung affections and pleurisy and for promoting the digestion and strengthening the nervous system.

Fomentations, Slap-on Compresses and Hot Rollers

Fomentations are useful chiefly for the relief of cramps, colics and aches. The wet-cloth is first soaked in warm water and, after folding, is heated in boiling water for a few minutes. It is pressed out by hand (well-protected), wrapped in a flannel cloth and then applied. The dry cloth and piece of woollen blanket are used to cover it and a hot water bottle is often laid on top of these to boost the effect.

Slap-on compresses consist of a piece of linen cloth wrapped round a wooden bar. This implement is dipped in boiling water and then *very briefly* pressed against the skin until it reddens. Slap-on compresses have proved themselves to be especially effective in cases of neuralgia.

For Hot Rollers a length of cloth is folded until its width is the same as that of the section of body to be treated. It is then rolled into a sort of funnel and hot water is poured into it. When all the layers of cloth are saturated, the 'funnel' is pressed together to make a roll and is applied to the skin. The advantage is obvious: as soon as the heat begins to dissipate, the roll is unrolled slightly until the next, still really hot, part is exposed. This enables one to obtain a particularly good, deep action.

Sacks and Cataplasms

The hayseed sack was one of Kneipp's favourite 'discoveries'. A linen sack, as large as the area to be treated, is two-thirds filled with hayseed, sewn up, and left to seethe for about 20 minutes in a pot of boiling water. It is then squeezed out between two boards under strong pressure and, as soon as its temperature has fallen to around 40°C/104°F, it is used as a body pack. Hayseed is recommended mainly for diseases of the joints, muscles and skin, for inflammations of the respiratory tract and colics in the digestive system. Pads of cotton wool are employed to protect the closed eyes before face applications are made.

Crushed linseed or potatoes cooked in their jackets are used in the same way as the hayseed, the potatoes being well mashed in the sack after cooking.

Linseed and fenugreek seed are also used for cataplasms. The crushed seeds are mixed with water and slowly cooked to a pap with constant stirring. The pap is spread in a finger-thick layer on the cloth and applied in the usual way.

CHAPTER 4

AFFUSIONS

Tap-cold water that is not under pressure is used for affusions. Only in exceptional circumstances will it be necessary to warm the water a little. In domestic practice, the rose is unscrewed from the bathroom shower and is replaced by a rubber tube about 2cm (¾ inch) thick. The rose itself is unsuitable for affusions as it does not deliver the necessary sheet of water.

When the mouth of the tube is pointing upwards, the jet of water should rise to about a hands-breadth. The mouth of the tube is always held 5-10cm (2-4 ins) from the body and is kept pointing downwards. It is important that a closed sheet of water is formed on the skin which, in a few minutes, will react by reddening, so producing a feeling of warmth.

When the affusion is over, the water is wiped off superficially and the patient goes to bed or dresses quickly and by keeping on the move will warm up and dry off fairly quickly.

Water jets can be utilized only with an experienced helper. In these, the water strikes the skin at two to three times atmosphere pressure from a distance of 4m (13ft), so that the effect is due not only to the temperature difference but also to the mechanical pressure involved.

The mouth of the tube should have a 0.5cm (¼-inch) diameter opening. Ideally it should be fitted with a 10cm (4 inch) long steel tube, so that the nurse, by placing her finger on its tip, can reduce the discharge or make it spurt out as she requires.

N.B. Always wear a rubber apron or some other form of waterproof clothing when experimenting with jets of water.

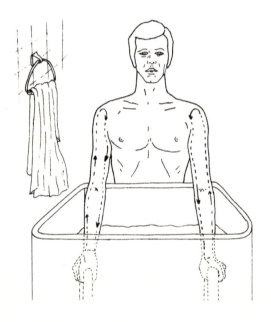

Fig. 9. Arm Affusion

The Arm Affusion
Ideally, the patient leans over some form of framework to support his arms. The right side is treated first, starting from the back of the hand and following the outside of the arm up to the shoulder. The water is allowed to play

on this spot for 10 seconds and is then brought down to the hand again. The left arm is treated in the same way. After the outsides of the arms have been well doused, their insides are treated similarly.

The Knee Affusion
In the knee affusion the back of the right foot is first exposed to a stream of water played backwards and forwards over it three times. The stream is then carried up over the outer calf as far as the knee-hollow, where there is a 10 second wait. It is then returned to the foot via the inside of the shin. With the left leg, the procedure is the same as far as the knee-hollow, but from there the stream of water is moved across horizontally to touch the right leg. It is allowed to stay there for a few seconds and is

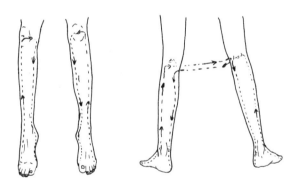

Fig. 10. Knee Affusion and Jet Treatment

then brought back across and slowly returned to the left foot down the inside of the left leg. In front, the affusion is again started at the outside of the right foot. It is carried up to the knee, is left there for a short time and then brought down again on the inside. The front of the left leg is treated in the same manner. The reaction (reddening, a feeling of warmth) can be obtained only from the musculature; care is taken, therefore, not to treat the shin-bone directly, since not only would this accomplish nothing but is rather painful.

Leg Affusion
Leg affusions are 'extended' knee affusions. This means that they are carried up to the hip on the outside of the leg. One starts with the back of the right leg as in the knee affusion. On the left one waits at hip height for the commencement of the reaction (reddening, a feeling of warmth) then turns to the right below the buttocks where there is another pause for the reaction. The stream of water is then carried down on the inner side of the leg back to the foot. In front, the affusion is taken up as far as the groin, but the bladder and abdomen must be left untouched. After a reaction has set in, one crosses over from left to right at mid-thigh level, returning to the left after a further reaction and carries the affusion down to the foot again as in the knee affusion.

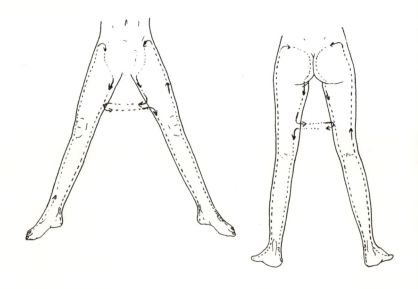

Fig. 11. Leg Affusion

Face Affusion
Face affusions are suitable for treating dirty skin and for
headaches and toothaches. The treatment starts below
the right temple, is taken down to the chin and back up to
the forehead. The forehead is then treated from right to
left horizontally and the water is passed over the rest of
the face in long strokes and, to finish, the water is moved
round the face in an oval direction.

Head Affusion
Head affusions begin behind the right ear and are taken
round in a large circle passing over the left ear and the
forehead. The stream of water is carried upwards over the
head in ever-decreasing circles until it reaches the crown
and is then taken back in the same way. The hair must be
very thoroughly dried after this treatment. This is most
important.

Upper Body Affusion
The patient, as in the arm affusion, bends over a support.
The application starts on the inside of the right arm, goes
up to the shoulder and returns to the wrist. Continuing
now with the left arm, the affusion is carried up along the
inside as far as the arm-pit and from there is moved over
the chest in a big circle or, in the case of women is moved
round the breasts in a figure-of-eight. From just below
the right breast, the stream is taken round to the back. At
the same time the patient must take a deep breath.
    Finally, the water is played on the right and left halves
of the back from top to bottom by using circling move-
ments. This application is chiefly used to aid the heart and
lungs.

Back Affusion
The whole back of the body is treated in this affusion. It
starts on the outside of the right foot, rises as far as the hip
and returns down the inside of the leg. On the left, the
treatment rises to hip level in the same way but returns
over and round the left buttock only as far as the top
inside of the thigh. From there it moves up diagonally
under the right buttock to the right elbow and up to
shoulder level. Here there is a pause of a few seconds
before the affusion is carried straight down the back to

the top of the right thigh again. After another sweeping movement, under the left buttock and up the left arm to the shoulder, the stream of water is carried straight down the left-hand side of the back, over the left buttock and down the inside of the left leg to the foot. Finally, each half of the back is given a dousing twice, the change-over from one side to the other being made under the buttocks. Water must not be directed at the spine itself. During treatment the patient breathes deeply and regularly, and the chest and back are splashed with cold water before the affusion commences to prepare the body for the shock.

Before a back affusion is undertaken, the doctor must be consulted, as this treatment is not tolerated by everybody.

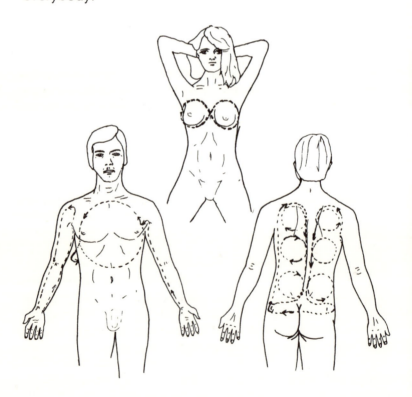

Fig. 12. Upper Body Affusion

Lower Body Affusion

The lower body affusion is similar to the leg affusion except that at the back it rises above the hips and buttocks to the waist and, at the front, it rises to the costal arch (immediately below the ribs). The intention is to form a closed sheet of water over the body and legs.

The Full Affusion

The full affusion starts at the outside of the right foot, is carried up to the hip and then down again on the inside of the leg. The left leg is treated in the same way as far as hip level and then the stream of water is moved over and round the left buttock, underneath the right buttock, across the tops of the thighs, and up the right arm to the shoulder. Here there is a pause of several seconds to allow a sheet of water to be formed on the right-hand side of the body (mainly on the back itself). The stream is returned straight down the back to the right thigh and then taken across to and up the left arm in a similar manner. It is zig-zagged from side to side over the neck a few times and, when the reaction has set in, is carried down the left-hand side of the back, over the buttocks and down the inside of the left leg to the foot.

The nurse now faces the patient from the front, starting with the right arm and moving up to the shoulder, where a sheet of water is once more allowed to form, this time over the front of the body. The affusion is taken downwards to the base of the trunk, carried across the tops of the thighs and up the opposite arm to the left shoulder, from where it is zig-zagged from side to side several times over the breast-bone (sternum). Finally it is brought down the left side again.

Full affusions have a very powerful action and should, therefore, never be attempted without the doctor's permission, or before the body has been hardened with partial affusions.

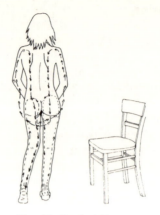

Fig. 13. Back Affusion

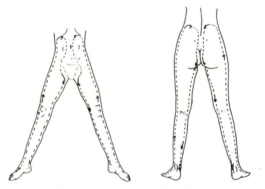

Fig. 14. Lower Body Affusion

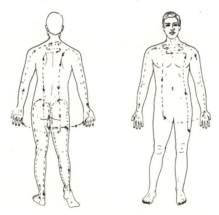

Fig. 15. Full Affusions

CHAPTER 5

JETS

Knee Jet and Leg Jet

Knee jets and leg jets start with a spray which is lifted from foot to knee-hollow or up to the buttocks, after which the full force of the water-jet is applied up the right calf until it is over the knee-hollow or buttocks and is then carried down the leg again to the heel. In leg jets the stream of water is circled round the buttock three times. The left leg is treated in exactly the same way and, finally, the water is splashed up and down both legs or calves. The patient now turns to face the nurse, who carries the jet of water up the front of his right leg and circles it in the region of his groin three times (but not directly on the crotch of course), or, in the case of the knee-jet treatment, circulates the water round his knee in the same way. Avoiding the shin-bone, she returns the jet to the foot via the inside of his leg. The left leg is given the same treatment.

Next, the water is splashed up and down the fronts of both legs exactly as was done on their backs. Finally, the patient turns side-on to the nurse, who treats the outside of his right leg or calf with the jet at full strength, and the inside of his left leg or calf at reduced pressure. The outside of the left leg and the inside of the right leg are then similarly treated. After this the soles of his feet are treated and finally the patient slowly turns round while his legs are covered with a fine spray.

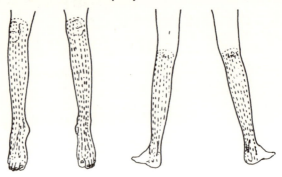

Fig. 16. Knee Jet

Full Jet

Like the full affusion, the full jet must be used only after the body has been inured to partial applications of the same kind and never without the doctor's permission. First of all, the back of the body is sprayed from feet to shoulders. Next the jet is played on the backs of the legs as in the leg-jet treatment. Then the jet is taken up the right arm as far as the shoulder-blade, is circled round the latter three times and brought down the inside of the arm to be crossed to the other arm at thigh-top level. The procedure is then repeated on the left-hand side. Then the water-jet crosses the middle of the thigh to the right side of the back and is swept in long strokes from the buttock to the shoulder.

After the left-hand side of the back has been treated in the same manner, the jet is played up and down the whole back by zig-zagging it from side to side, and is finally brought down the left leg to the foot. The treatment of the back is concluded by spraying the arms and legs up and down.

The patient now turns to face the nurse, who moves the jet of water over his legs and loins. The jet is then taken up the outside of the right arm and circled round the right breast three times. It is brought down the same arm, on the inside, passed across the middle of the thighs to

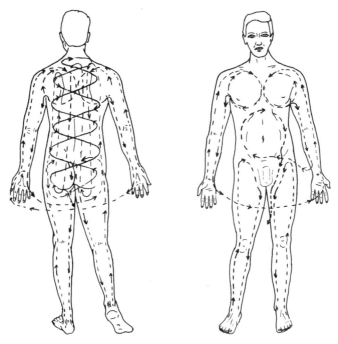

Fig. 17. Full Jet

the left arm. The left breast is also circled three times but, when the jet is played down the inside of the left arm, it is circled around the abdomen at reduced pressure. The jet is then taken down over the left leg. Finally, the patient turns side-on to the nurse with his arms raised above his head and one leg in front of the other, while she plays the water-jet over him from his feet up to his arm-pit. Finally, she treats the soles of his feet and gives him a shower over his whole body.

Because it is obvious that water jetting under pressure is liable to make a mess, this type of treatment should not be undertaken without proper preparations. It would be best to have the use of a large tiled bathroom with floor plumbing to carry away the waste water, even though a certain amount of good may be done with the patient standing in the bath. The home nurse should also take the precaution of wearing a long rubber apron or overall to avoid a soaking.

CHAPTER 6

BATHS

A bath, even when used simply for cleansing the body, can be too strong a stimulus for a feeble or sickly person. Therefore its application in a major way as, for example, in the form of a complete bath, a half bath or a hip bath, will always require the doctor's permission. Hot baths are frequently employed with additives such as oatstraw, pine needles, camomile, horsetail and similar ingredients. Below are some of the medical recommendations. The dose is the usual one for domestic treatments and the stated amounts are for a complete bath:

Bath Additives
Valerian. Use the tincture as directed on the bottle or infuse 100g (4 oz) of the dried herb in 1 litre (about 2 pints) water. Indicated in nervousness and sleep disorders.
Pine needles. Use the pine oil as directed on the bottle or make a decoction of 1kg (2 lbs) pine needles and pine cones. Indicated in nervousness, sleep disorders, neuralgia and rheumatism.
Oat straw. Make a decoction of 1 wisp of straw in 1 large pot of water. Indicated in skin diseases, rheumatism and gout.

Camomile. Use 100g (4 oz) flower heads as an infusion. Indicated in haemorrhoids (piles) and skin diseases.

Lavender. Make a decoction of 100g (4 oz) flower spikes. Indicated as a stimulus in nervous diseases and for nervous disorders in general.

Rosemary. Make an infusion of 50g (2 oz) leaves. Indicated in nervous disorders and especially in heart trouble, low blood pressure and rheumatism. Never use at night.

Horsetail. Prepare 150g (5 oz) in 5 litres (9 pints) water as an infusion. Indicated in rheumatism, gout and skin diseases.

Note. In an infusion, boiling water is poured over the herbs and they are left to steep as in making tea whereas, in a decoction the herbs are boiled to extract their active principles.

Complete Bath

Hot baths last about 15 minutes. They are soothing and relaxing and therefore aid sleep, they also promote elimination via the skin. After the bath, a cold shower is taken or a quick dip in cold water.

Graduated baths start with the temperature of the water at 35°C/95°F and are then slowly topped up with hot water until a temperature of 39-41°C (102-106°F) is reached. These baths relieve cramps and improve the circulation. The bath is ended as soon as perspiration commences. Afterwards, the patient has a cold wash or works off his perspiration in bed.

Contrast baths begin in hot water, where the patient remains for five minutes. He then changes to a cold bath for 15 seconds, returns to the hot bath and, finally, gets back into the cold water again. Contrast baths are usually given as partial applications to patients with weak reactions. The cold-water baths last only 5 to 20 seconds and end as soon as a warm reaction or painful ache is felt.

Generally speaking, a complete contrast bath cannot be taken at home. Not many domestic bathrooms are equipped with the necessary twin tubs. One can take a quick cold shower between two soaks in the full hot bath, but this is only a makeshift solution. It is recommended that a cold bath be taken on rising from bed, while the body is still warm and, when the dip is over, that exercise be taken to warm up again. Such baths, which make considerable demands on the stamina, act on the nerves, the metabolism and the circulation.

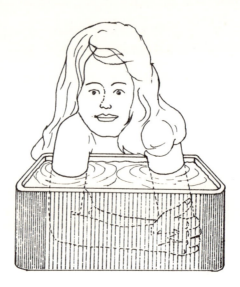

Fig. 18. Arm Bath

The Arm Bath
This reaches to just below the shoulders and should be taken if possible with both arms submerged at the same time. Cold arm baths last for not more than half a minute. To avoid shock, the arms are lowered in slowly. As soon as the reaction (reddening, a sensation of warmth) sets in, the arms are scrubbed or swung round to warm them up. Hot arm baths last for up to 20 minutes and end with a short cold dip or affusion. The graduated arm bath should be raised from 35°C/95°F to 41°C/106°F in 10 minutes. Arm baths influence the heart, improve the circulation and relieve cramps and inflammations of the finger, lymph vessels and joints.

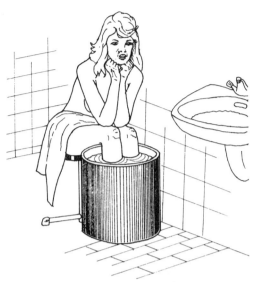

Fig. 19. Foot Bath

Foot Bath and Lower-leg Bath
Owing to the influence of the local dialect in Kneipp's part of Germany, 'foot bath' has come to mean a bath that reaches above mid-calf level. The illustration shows the size of tub required (for contrast baths, two tubs will be required, of course). For want of better, a large pail would service.

Cold foot baths, for strengthening and to alleviate sleep disorders, last only a few seconds, until the reaction begins. The contrast foot bath, which is used for poor circulation, foot disorders (flat feet, etc.) and various disorders of the abdomen, kidneys and bladder, begins with hot water, is changed to a quick dip in cold water and then back to hot water again. This is done three times in all, ending with a cold dip.

Graduated foot baths (35°C/95°F-41°C/106°F) which are used for kidney, bladder and respiratory diseases, for rheumatism, gout and arteriosclerosis, are ended as soon as perspiration commences. The patient then retires to bed to work off his perspiration for 1 hour before the treatment is concluded with a cold affusion.

Hot foot baths, of about 39°C/102°F and lasting 15 minutes, are recommended for podobromidrosis (strong-smelling perspiration of the feet) and for cold feet. Horsetail, woodashes, salt and various other medicinal herbs form suitable additives.

Eye Bath and Face Bath
In both baths, a sufficiently large bowl is required for immersing the face completely. In the eye bath, the eyes are opened under water several times. The face is lifted out of the water to take breath three times. For acute diseases of the eyes, warm eye baths with the addition of extract of euphrasia (eyebright), fennel or horsetail plant can be used, but only with the permission of an oph-thalmologist. The practitioner's instructions must be exactly observed. It is especially important to make sure that the eyewash contains no solid residues when additives are employed, so that they do not get into the eyes. Cold baths are particularly useful for strengthening the eyes.

The cold or hot face bath, with camomile and horsetail, is an important cleanser of dirty facial skin.

Hip Bath
Hip baths are taken either in a special tub or in any other suitable tub. The water should reach to the level of the kidneys and should cover the mid-thighs. Cold hip baths last from 5 to 20 seconds and are carried out with the upper body clothed. In hot hip baths, which last for about 15 minutes, the patient and the tub are covered in sheets. The feet, which have been previously well-warmed, are placed on a low stool in front of the tub. The hot hip bath is ended with a short cold affusion or cold dip and a rest in bed. After the cold hip bath, it is necessary to warm up again quickly by taking exercise, after which the patient retires to bed to work off his perspiration.

Graduated hip baths can also be taken. Hip baths influence the abdominal urinary and digestive organs. They are indicated, for example, in cramps, gripping pains, swellings, obstructions (including constipation) and haemorrhoids (piles).

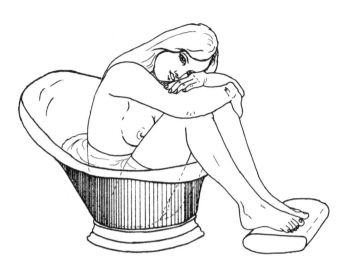

Fig. 20. Hip Bath

Half Baths

In half baths the water covers the body together with the legs up to the navel. Hot half baths replace the complete bath when the latter is not well tolerated. The graduated half bath is indicated in rheumatism and gout of the legs and hip-joints. Cold half baths of from 5 to 10 seconds duration are strengthening and alleviate sleep disorders and the troubles treated by hip baths. After the half bath, the same procedure is adopted as after the hip bath.

Complete Baths

Complete baths affect the whole body, which is submerged up to and over the shoulders. People with circulatory and cardiac diseases should not try this taxing treatment, at least not before the doctor has been consulted. Hot complete baths are usually employed with additives. There is also the hyperthermal bath, which is always taken under professional supervision. Cold baths of this sort last no more than a few seconds; hot complete baths take from 15 to 20 minutes. At the end of a complete bath, the same procedure is followed as was explained in the section on the hip bath.

CHAPTER 7

VAPOUR TREATMENTS

These hot applications last for from 10 to 30 minutes. They warm the body passively, the peripheral circulation is improved and so is the general circulation and the metabolism. The reaction sought is free perspiration, even in those parts of the body which have not been exposed to the vapour. The action is improved by the use of additives as in the hot baths. Three handfuls of the herbs are boiled for half an hour in a covered vessel, care being taken that the pot is not filled too high as that would hinder the development of the vapour. The lid is gradually slid open. As soon as the vapour production diminishes, more may be produced by cautiously putting a hot stone into the water. Care must be taken that the stone is slid into the water not dropped into it, otherwise scalding drops will be thrown out.

At the end of the application, the patient retires to bed to work off his perspiration, and as soon as the perspiration stops the treatment is concluded with a cold affusion. One must never go out into the open air immediately after a vapour treatment.

Vapour treatments are relaxing and should not be employed too often. Vapour treatments are to be distinguished from a steam bath in a bathroom or sauna.

Steam Bath

Steam baths taken in air saturated with water vapour at temperatures of around 50°C/122°F last for 10 minutes to begin with; later this can be increased to 20 minutes. The steam bath, which is also known as a turkish bath, is concluded with a cold shower or a cold complete bath. Steam baths are contraindicated (i.e. must *not* be taken) in high fevers, after eating and in cardiovascular diseases. They must never be used without the doctor's permission.

Sauna

The sauna is a hot-air bath taken in extremely dry air, in which temperatures of up to 95°C/203°F are reached and well tolerated. In principle, the doctor should always be consulted before resorting to saunas, which are not suited to cases of cardiac, circulatory and tubercular disease.

The indications for medical use are, just as in the steam bath, metabolic diseases, skin diseases and rheumatism. It is not merely the hot air which is effective in a sauna but also the alternation between hot and cold (cold complete bath, or treading in water or snow).

Never take a sauna on a full stomach. The best time for a visit is in the early evening. Usually, after 10 to 15 minutes in the hot atmosphere, a quick cold bath is taken and the whole process is repeated twice, a cold application being used to finish. This is followed by a rest of half an hour.

Vapour Bath for Head and Face

In both these forms of vapour application the vapour pot is placed on a chair or table and the patient sits in front of it. In the head treatment, the upper part of the body is undressed. A sheet is thrown over the upper body, vapour pot and table in such a way that no vapour can escape from underneath it. As the vapour rises it is breathed in deeply through the mouth and nose. Finally, the parts of the body treated are washed in cold water. It is indicated for unclean facial skin (add camomile or horsetail herb here for preference), inflammations of the nose, nasal sinuses, bronchial tubes and eyes and also for ulcers or eczemas in those parts of the body exposed to the vapour.

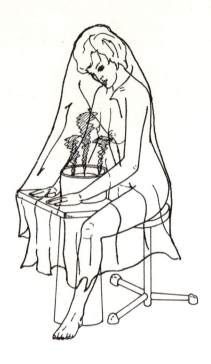

Fig. 21. Vapour Bath for Head and Face

Vapour Bath for the Feet

This is indicated in feet suffering from chronic coldness or excessive perspiration. The patient sits, with the lower body unclothed, on a chair the seat of which is covered with a woollen blanket with a linen sheet on top. A covered vapour pot is placed in front of the feet. The lower body and pot are enveloped in the sheets, care being taken that there is a good seal at the bottom to prevent any escape of vapour. The nurse now slowly uncovers the pot, puts a framework of wooden slats across it and gets the patient to place his feet on it. The treatment ends with a cold wash.

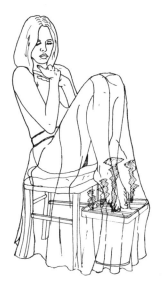

Fig. 22. Vapour Bath for Feet

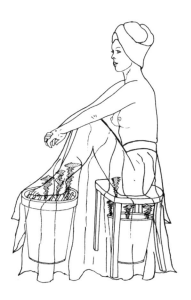

Fig. 23. Half Vapour Bath

Half Vapour Bath

Both of these vapour baths require a chair with an open-work seat to allow the vapour through to the patient. The lower body is undressed but the upper body remains clothed. The covers reach from the floor to the hips and

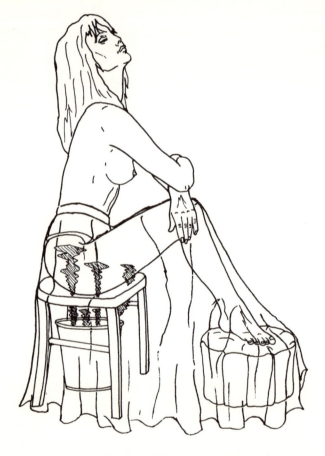

Fig. 24. Lower Body Vapour Bath

envelop not only the seat of the chair but the entire chair, which is a point of difference between them and the vapour bath for the feet.

In the half vapour bath the patient sits with his chair over one vapour pot and his feet resting on an open wooden frame on top of a second pot as in the vapour bath for the feet.

The lower body vapour bath differs from the half vapour bath in that the feet are not placed over a second vapour pot but are well warmed and placed on the floor.

Half vapour baths and lower body vapour baths are useful in diseases of the abdominal organs, urinary tracts and liver, for abdominal colics and for menstrual disorders.

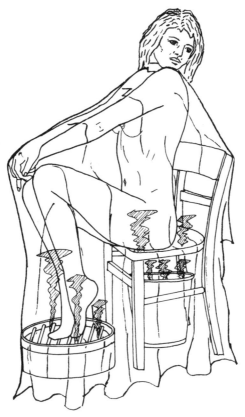

Fig. 25. Complete Vapour Bath

Complete Vapour Bath
In complete vapour baths, the vapour pots, as in the half vapour bath, are placed beneath a chair with an open-

work seat and also under the feet. The wrapping sheets, however, are tucked in at the neck to form a good seal and envelop the whole body together with the chair and the pots. They rest on the floor all the way round to prevent any vapour escaping. Complete vapour baths are indicated when the patient is not able to tolerate a steam bath. They last for 10 minutes only, after which the patient goes to bed for a while to work off his perspiration and finally takes a cold dip or a cold affusion.

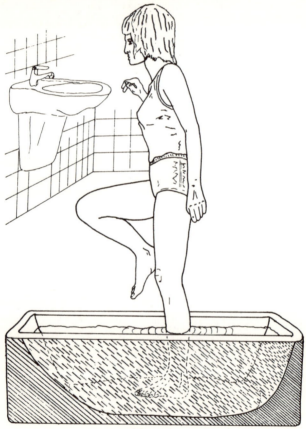

Fig. 26. Water Treading

Water Treading

Water treading lasts for about two minutes. The reaction is either a pleasant warm glow in the feet or a sharp ache that is followed by warmth. Given the opportunity, it is a good idea to tread water in a brook with the water coming to mid-calf level. However, it is also possible to step up and down in the domestic bath-tub filled with cold water.

Walking barefoot through the snow has been found useful in winter. Care must be taken, however, to avoid snow on which a crust has formed, otherwise the feet may be hurt.

Finally, there is the possibility of running through dew-covered or even dry grass, although one must not expect a reaction until three to four minutes have elapsed.

Kneipp made a special point of recommending walking in water, dew or snow as strengthening activities. They have a value in insomnia, too, although the wet sock treatment or foot baths will often be preferred as more convenient.

Dispersion and Activation
All water treatments are either dispersive or activating. Dispersion means removing a plethora or stasis of blood, such as can occur in an inflamed part of the body, and taking the surplus to some other part of the body. Compresses, affusions and baths are suitable for this purpose. There are rules for dispersion between different parts of the body, as follows: from the head to the chest, arms and legs; from the chest to the arms and legs; from the body to the legs; and from the legs to the arms or to the body.

For example, dispersion in the arms and legs is carried out by means of arm baths, foot baths, arm compresses, calf compresses, wet socks, treading in water, dew and snow, arm affusions, leg and knee affusions. In the body, dispersion is brought about by the use of short compresses and loin compresses, hip baths and half baths, and in the chest by means of chest compresses and shawls.

Activation affects the skin, the secretory organs, kidneys and intestines. Compresses and other diaphoretic applications are given preference for activation of the skin.

CHAPTER 8

GYMNASTICS AND SPORT

During Kneipp's lifetime, gymnastics were over-emphasized in schools and had too limited a range. His scepticism on the subject of sport was therefore partly justified. Nowadays, on the other hand, physical education is considered less important and Kneipp would have been glad that the schools offer as much as they do.

Kneipp's critical attitude to physical education did not imply a rejection of bodily exercise. On the contrary, he was always advocating the use of sensible exercise both in everyday life and as part of a course of treatments. However, he set more store by real hard manual work. Today, machines are taking it more and more off our hands and we need something like digging in the garden or allotment to offset this loss.

Type of Sport
The choice of sport will depend, first of all, on personal preference. There should be no compulsory sets of exercises and no striving for attainment. Most of us operate under many pressures in our daily lives and are faced with competitors and the need to do well; surely, there is no need to import all this stress into our free time. The individual who trains doggedly merely to achieve

something is not doing his health any good. The best plan is to enjoy some form of physical recreation with family, friends or colleagues in a relaxed, friendly atmosphere. The possibility of social contact, missed by so many in everyday life, will then be added to the benefits of bodily exercise.

To put it in a nutshell: taking exercise should be fun and it must be adapted to the physical capacity of the individual. Sports doctors recommend exercising the body once a day to the extent that the pulse beat per minute reaches 180 minus the age in years. According to this rule-of-thumb, an organically healthy person at the age of 40 should reach a pulse rate of 140 per minute. The doctor should, of course, be consulted before any sort of exercise is taken up.

Bad weather is no excuse for foregoing a day's exercise in the open air. There is no risk to health in venturing out of doors in the most inclement weather provided the appropriate clothing is worn. It is desirable that at least one hour should be spent every day in this way.

Swimming, walking and light gymnastics are suitable for people of almost any age and constitution. Long cycle rides, skiing or cross-country running are not for everybody. Personal preference and physical capacity enter into the question of horse-racing, water-skiing, mountaineering, football, golf, dancing and many other forms of exercise.

The Daily Dozen
On rising in the morning and in the evening before going to bed, 5 to 10 minutes should be spent in simple exercises in front of an open window—even in winter. Breaks during the day should be utilized for performing compensatory exercises to forestall damage due to a onesided stressing of the body during working hours. Even when one is under great pressure to finish an urgent job, the few minutes spent in this manner will not be wasted, because efficiency will be noticeably improved.

Special remedial exercises for specific diseases, on the other hand, must always be performed under the guidance of a trained instructor, otherwise they will do more harm than good.

Breathing Exercises

The nervous disorders so common today can be influenced by a special form of exercise, that is, by breathing exercises. Faulty breathing threatens to become a 'plague' in all the industrialized nations. Our hectic life-style is leading more and more to quick, shallow breathing with all its disadvantages.

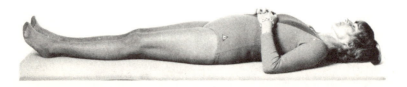

Fig. 27. Abdominal Breathing

Breathing exercises train the breathing in such a way that, in the end, the individual breathes correctly without even realizing it. Nevertheless, because there are many illnesses in which breathing exercises are forbidden, the doctor must always be consulted before starting to do them. Often he will want to make sure they are being done properly, too. As a remedial measure, breathing exercises must always be performed under professional supervision.

When doing breathing exercises, one preferably lies loose and relaxed on the bed or on a flat board that is raised 20 to 40cms (8-16 ins) at the foot according to the exercise. To begin with, only abdominal respiration is used (neglected above all by women). Then the person breathes out as much as possible, so that the abdomen and chest both sink in visibly. After that as deep a breath as can be managed is taken, so that the abdomen can be seen to arch up. A heavy book resting on the abdomen will strengthen the action.

After abdominal breathing has been mastered, costal respiration (respiration based mainly on the rib-cage) is practised. In principle, this is similar to abdominal breathing. First of all, there is maximal expiration, then a breath is taken deep enough to raise the chest visibly. Finally, costal and abdominal breathing are performed together. Deep abdominal breathing is used first and then, during the same in-breath, there is a change-over to deep costal breathing. In the second phase of costal-breathing the level of the abdomen drops a little. Expiration commences at the abdomen and then the chest surface is allowed to fall.

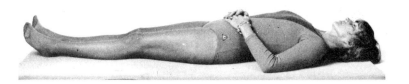

Fig. 28. Costal Breathing

In each form of breathing the ratio of inspiration to expiration is 1 to 2. Hence breathing out takes twice as long as breathing in. Between the end of expiration and renewed inspiration there is a pause, which should last three times as long as the time taken by the inspiration. Even the deepest inhalation is always made through the nose; expiration meets resistance from the closed lips, which may cause a slight humming perhaps. Such breathing exercises are useful not only for influencing the respiratory organs and the heart and circulation or for bringing about a natural respiratory rhythm but also they form a prelude to the various relaxation exercises and are a part of Hatha Yoga. As a rule, ten complete breaths are taken per exercise.

Photos taken from the book *Schlank nach Plan* (Planned Slimming) published by Walter Hädecke Verlag.

CHAPTER 9

AIR AND SUN BATHS

Open-air Baths
Air baths in the open are employed as rest cures or as part of a health programme involving outdoor games and sport, but hot sunlight and draughts are avoided. The body is adjusted to this by, initially taking an air bath, unclothed, in a heated room. Gradual modifications are then introduced, starting with the use of an unheated room and continuing with opening a window in the unheated room until the individual is ready to take an air bath out of doors. After some practice, an open-air bath can even be taken in sub-zero conditions without any danger to health. Their duration will depend on the weather but, on average, they will not exceed two thirty-minute periods daily. When outside temperatures are low, these baths must occupy considerably less time of course.

Open-air baths stimulate the metabolism, the body's defences, the endocrine glands, the circulation and the nervous system.

Sun Baths
A person must accustom himself or herself to sunbathing too, otherwise there is a risk of skin damage.

On the first day only the feet and lower legs are exposed, front and back, to the sun for five minutes each. On the following day the exposure is increased to ten minutes and the upper leg is also uncovered. On the third day the bath lasts for ten minutes again on each side of the body, and the abdomen is also exposed to the sun. It is not before the fourth day that the back is also sunned for ten minutes. On the fifth day the whole body is given a sun bath on the front and back for fifteen minutes each and, as the treatment progresses from day to day, the exposure to the rays of the sun is slowly increased up to one hour at a time.

Sun baths are taken in a place that is sheltered from the wind and, in summer, in the early morning before the heat of the day. The head and neck are protected with a hat or scarf and the eyes by means of sunglasses. In the beginning, when only part of the body is being treated the parts not being so treated can easily be covered with a towel. As soon as the stage is reached where the whole body can be exposed to sunlight, the individual no longer lies stewing in the heat but keeps on the move, seeking the cool shade from time to time. Sunbathing may be done out of doors even in the colder seasons when the sunshine is much less strong and makes its appearance more briefly, provided that the body has already been inured in the way described above. Those who sun themselves under glass in a covered veranda or other type of glazed interior will be disappointed in the effect. Ordinary window glass admits hardly any ultra-violet light. Special panes have to be put in for that purpose. On dull days a sun-lamp may be used but, if at all possible, one should enjoy the natural sunlight.

Sunbathing stimulates the metabolism, the body's natural defences and the nervous system, and benefit skin diseases and other disorders.

CHAPTER 10

A WELL-BALANCED DIET

The Rev. Kneipp was never one-sided in his approach, even on the subject of right feeding. He recommended no special diet but rather a sensible, coarse diet of everything offered to us by Nature—provided some organic disease does not place certain restrictions on our feeding. He neither condemned nor recommended meat-eating but suggested that flesh be used with moderation. Kneipp was far ahead of his time in this respect, for it is only recently that research carried out at the Max Planck Institute, Dortmund has refuted the widespread belief that it is flesh alone that provides the full range of proteins our bodies require. This research has shown that any mixture of several protein foods has more value than a single protein food eaten on its own. The highest value is possessed by a combination of eggs and potato protein, next in order come eggs and wheat, then milk and bread, and only in fourth place do we find the combination of meat and potatoes.

Kneipp's mixed diet contained a lot of roughage to regulate the bowels. This is especially important today, since an increasing number of people, notably women, complain of constipation. Fruit, vegetables and salad plants should be eaten raw if possible, as it is only when fresh and uncooked that they retain their vital elements in full strength. Kneipp considered that curdled milk, buttermilk and curds were particularly valuable articles of diet. This opinion of his has been confirmed by modern food science. Meat and meat products should be eaten no more than once a day; eggs, salt and condiments (except pot herbs) should be used sparingly. What is more, one should cut down on, or better still cut out, all fatty meats, sausages and fish, particularly pork, bacon, ham, eels, duck, goose and pickled herring or corned beef, also all kinds of tinned and ready-cooked foods, blancmange, semolina, refined products like white flour, white sugar and other denatured foods.

The food ought to be prepared with a view to preserving as much of its goodness as possible; therefore it is better grilled and stewed than it is boiled and roasted. Books are readily available from the shops for anyone interested in the principles of preparing healthy meals that will provide a well-balanced diet. It would take us too far afield at the present time to give general advice based on modern nutrition research together with detailed applications and recipes. However, a fair idea of what is meant by a well-balanced diet may be gained from the following specimen menu for guests taking the cure in Bad Wörishofen. Anyone who adopts it will be assured of a well-balanced diet which will maintain health and energy.

Balanced Menu
Breakfast
Crispbread and all kinds of wholemeal bread.
Butter or vegetable oil margarine.
Jam or honey.
Muesli (Bircher's muesli) or fresh fruit.
Ordinary coffee or caffeine-free coffee.
Malted milk, plain milk, Indian tea, herb-tea, or fruit juice.

Midday Meal
Fruit and vegetable juices, uncooked food, salad, vegetable soup.
Lean meat and non-fatty fish, poultry, eggs.

Potatoes (boiled, in their jackets or mashed), rice, wholemeal products, farinaceous food.

Vegetables according to the time of year and as desired.

Fruit.

Evening Meal

Wholemeal bread and crispbread.

Butter, buttermilk, curdled milk, yourt, curds.

Low-fat cheese.

Uncooked food, mixed salads.

Advice on eating can be obtained at all health food stores.

If one is not on any special diet, and after due consultation with the doctor, fast-days may be observed from time to time, or days on which fruit or fruit juice or vegetables or rice or potatoes form the sole items of diet. The purpose of this is detoxication, drainage and regulation of the metabolism generally. Weekends are especially useful here.

Eating Correctly

It is not enough simply to eat the right things, the way one eats is equally important. Basically, one should eat only until one feels pleasantly satisfied, without having a sense of fullness or remaining hungry. As children, many of us were told to finish everything on our plates. This is something we should forget as quickly as possible, as it is the first step towards becoming overweight. A guilty conscience over leaving food on one's plate can be prevented by not taking so much in the first place—it is always possible to ask for a second helping if still hungry.

Eating should be enjoyable, indeed it should be a pleasure. For this it is essential to eat slowly and in a calm frame of mind, without having to watch the time and without being distracted by problems, or having one's nose buried in the newspaper. A relaxed atmosphere should always prevail when we are at the table and nothing should be allowed to spoil it. Problems and cares are better kept for some other time.

Thorough mastication is half the battle as far as digestion is concerned, for as the mouthful is mechanically broken up it is well-mixed with the saliva and so prepared for further disintegration lower down. Proper chewing is also important for dental health. The work involved in dealing with coarse food effectively inhibits caries. The most suitable form of mastication is known as Fletcherism, after the American Horace Fletcher (1848-1919) who introduced it to the public. In this system the food is so well masticated and mixed with saliva that by the time it is swallowed it is almost completely fluid.

Beverages

Kneipp was not radically opposed to people's favourite beverages. He believed with Paracelsus that, 'it is only the size of the dose that decides whether something is a poison or not'. Taken in reasonable amounts, there is no objection to a glass of wine or beer or a cup of coffee, provided no organic disease makes their use unwise. But pleasant beverages should be no more than just that; when they are a simple pleasure and nothing else, they can do no harm. However, the person who drinks wine, beer and other alcoholic beverages by force of habit, or is one of today's social drinkers, or seeks to drown his sorrows in drink, has become an alcoholic even though he might hotly deny it. And the person who misuses the stimulant drug caffeine in coffee (or the related theine in strong tea) to overcome that feeling of tiredness which is warning him his body needs to rest, will quickly find that he has drained his energy reserves.

No Nicotine

The position is quite different with that poisonous pleasure, nicotine. Researches carried out in the recent past have so unequivocally exposed the risks to health run by the cigarette smoker in particular, that the strongest warning must be given against smoking tobacco. It is true enough that many folk simply enjoy an after-dinner cigar, an occasional pipe at the end of the day or a cigarette when they want to unwind and leave it at that, but if this is all they ask of tobacco then they should give it up completely. That may sound like a paradox, but at this stage it is still easy to wean themselves off the habit. As soon as the full addiction takes a hold with all its side-effects on the heart, circulation, respiratory tract, nervous system and indeed on the whole body, not forgetting the high risk of getting cancer run by smokers, it is very difficult to break free from it without relapsing. The best thing is to renounce smoking when one is young. Therefore all smoking parents should consider the effect their example is having on their uncritical children.

And now a word on smoking in women. When, in the aftermath of the Second World War, women took to cigarettes in a big way as part of their emancipation, they laid themselves open to the rapidly increasing incidence of lung cancer we see among them today. It can hardly be termed women's lib., in the true sense of the word, if all it means is the liberty to die in the same numbers as men from this terrible scourge. What is more, it shows an irresponsible attitude towards unborn life when women smoke during pregnancy

Basic Rules
Kneipp's views on feeding and our little indulgences in food and drink can be summed up in a few sentences, and are easy for every one to follow in daily life without going to any expense:
1. Do not eat meat products more than once a day.
2. If possible, do not eat tinned and other denatured foods. Eat only what is bought fresh, and make a regular practice of serving this fresh food uncooked.
3. A healthy, mixed and unrefined diet, offers the best guarantee of optimum nourishment.
4. An eighth or a quarter of a litre bottle of wine (one quarter to half a pint, approx.) or one or two glasses of beer a day are permissible. According to the researches of Prof. Schettler, one of Germany's best known specialists in internal medicine and heart disorders at the University of Heidelberg, small amounts of alcohol are not only allowable but are even beneficial. Although the full details have not yet been worked out, it looks as if there is a definite connection between the drinking of small amounts of alcohol and

a reduction in the risk of cardiac infarction (destruction of heart tissue due to blockage of the blood supply). The elderly can improve their sociability and their powers of attention with a moderate daily intake of alcohol. However, it must be borne in mind that alcohol is a source of calories and must not be left out of the picture when the rest of the diet is considered. The best advice is this: if you drink a lot give it up; if you drink a little still drink a little; if you don't drink, don't start.

5. Two or three cups of coffee per day will not hurt a healthy constitution. The morning cup can even prove beneficial to those with poor circulations. Use only pure ground coffee.

6. Spirits and fortified alcoholic drinks and nicotine should be avoided.

The man or woman who observes these rules will do what is needed to supply his body with the 'right building stones', as Kneipp used to say, for construction or repair.

PART THREE

MEDICAL INDICATIONS

CHAPTER 11

VEGETATIVE AND MENTAL DISORDERS

The number of the mentally ill is constantly rising today. In most instances our way of life is to blame, as it becomes less sensible and less in harmony with our natural needs. Apparently, we have not yet recovered from the jolting leap forward taken by civilization over two centuries ago at the time of the industrial revolution.

In all industrialized countries, doctors, psychologists and sociologists note with concern how people are becoming increasingly dependent on a form of technology designed to serve prestige-seekers and those who want to win the rat-race. They see people reduced to mere units in a consumer society. We are all constantly burdened and over-burdened by it. At the same time, by our refined living and our refined foods, we protect ourselves from the natural stimuli which would stiffen our powers of resistance.

Then there is a loss of the ability to speak with or listen to one another. The lack of communication between modern man and his fellows drives him still further into tormenting isolation and that baseless anxiety being found everywhere by medical observers.

This response of the soul to an environment that has grown hostile to man, will express itself partly on the level of the mind, as for example in eccentric behaviour, but partly too in disturbances of the fine adjustment of the vegetative nervous system and its associated organs. However, we would be exceeding the limits of this book if we were to go into the purely pscyhological symptoms involved. Of the functional phenomena that are responsive to the Kneipp Cure, we must distinguish between disturbances of vegetative sensibility and the ensuing multiple clinical picture of vegetative dystonia and nervousness.

Warning Signs

Initially there are unpleasant physical sensations whenever the tonicity of the vegetative nervous system adapts to changing situations. Usually we experience no more than occasional episodes such as, for example, a sudden sensation of falling, a shaking of the limbs or an indefinite queasy feeling. It is only when these things begin to intrude with increasing frequency, when zonaesthesia (the feeling of being constricted by a tight girdle) and a sense of pressure on the abdomen occur, when there is a sensation of a lump in the neck, with pains and feelings of tightness around the heart and cardiac palpitations, that we can speak of disturbances of the vegetative sensibility. The patients affected generally report that their troubles began insidiously and were accompanied by mental reactions. They almost invariably complain of anxiety. It is noticeable that quite slight stimuli, such as small disappointments, can lead to very passionate and explosive reactions, while a strong stimulus, even the death of a close acquaintance will provoke scarcely any reaction at all. This is all evidence that the state of the tonus has altered. People with jobs that demand thought and concentration complain more frequently than others do of this type of trouble. Only the specialist can say for certain whether the causes are vegetative or organic and decide on the treatment accordingly. 'Ignore it!' is the simplest advice to give in cases of vegetative disturbance, but that is too facile, since psychologically based suffering can be far more distressing than organic based suffering besides seriously alarming the patient about the state of his health.

Symptoms

Among the symptoms of vegetative dystonia are cardiac and respiratory troubles, insomnia, disorders of the digestive system, attacks of perspiration (especially damp cold hands), deafness, formication (a crawling sensation in the skin) in the limbs, giddiness, headache, restlessness and other symptoms. Strictly speaking, vegetative dystonia is not an illness but a symptom—of a neurosis for example. Many times it points to some organic deficiency such as anaemia and hormonal imbalance at puberty or with the menopause. However, in most instances the interplay of the sympathetic and parasympathetic systems is disturbed, in which event the close connection between the onset of the trouble and the mental life of the patient becomes evident.

Nervousness

Nervousness is the everyday term for a great number of health troubles similar to those of vegetative dystonia. This usage is not precise enough for doctors however. They understand it as a slight disturbance in control, in which adjustment to the environment is still fairly intact although it has become noticeably difficult, as evidenced by increased excitability and irritability and inner tension.

Nervousness can be a matter of temperament and is often seen in sensitive, creative people. Nevertheless it is often brought on by a life spent in unfavourable surroundings and by physical or mental diseases. Kneipp applications are very beneficial for the unpleasant bodily effects of vegetative and mental disturbances. Psychotherapy is frequently indicated as a supportive measure.

Sleep Disorders

When no organic causes, such as fever or pain, are present all dispersive measures are suitable. Of proved value are water treading out of bed, calf compresses, wet socks and foot baths. In addition, certain medicinal herbs are given, such as valerian, hops and balm. Bad habits such as general inactivity, eating poor food and other causes will have to be corrected. If the sleep disorders persist without any recognizable cause, a medical examination will be necessary.

Anxiety and Depression
Increased irritability and agitation can be due to temperament, to organic and mental illnesses or to unfavourable living conditions, overwork, noise, shift-work, the abuse of alcohol and nicotine, and unresolved conflicts. When the causes are organic and mental, medical advice must be sought. In other cases, especially where unfavourable conditions or temperament are concerned, dispersive measures such as arm and foot baths, wet socks, water treading, calf and loin compresses, short compresses and half baths with pine needles and lavender are indicated. In addition, valerian and hops are given and mistakes in the way of living are corrected as far as possible, perhaps through a change in dwelling or place of work or by giving up smoking or drinking or over-indulgence in strong tea or coffee.

Headache and Migraine
Any headaches which occur more frequently than or last longer than three days, must be checked by the doctor, because some organic disease may underlie them. Lesions of the vertebral column are frequent causes of headache, in which case an osteopath or chiropractor should be consulted.

Self-treatment with Kneipp applications is only for those occasional headaches from which we all suffer from time to time. Suitable water applications are treading in water and dew, contrast footbaths, knee and leg affusions, and half and hip baths. Cold compresses on the forehead and nape of the neck, are also useful. When the mind is disturbed, autogenic training and psychotherapy can be indicated. As supportive treatment, valerian, St John's wort, balm, peppermint, rosemary, and sage are given.

The diagnosis 'migraine' is for the specialist to make; too many other diseases simulate it for the layman to be sure. The same dispersive measures as in headache are indicated as a treatment.

In addition, it is helpful to drink strong black coffee with lemon juice or valerian, fennel, St John's Wort, camomile and marjoram tisanes.

A sensible life-style is particularly important, the avoidance of alcohol and nicotine etc., lots of exercise in the open air and the avoidance of constant stress.

Sensitivity to Weather

All the strengthening measures of the Kneipp System are suitable for sensitivity to weather. For example air baths, exercise in the open air and water treading. Valerian and hop tea are given in addition and, if the circulation is poor, a cup of coffee once in a while. Those who are sensitive to weather should visit the doctor for regular check-ups, as their trouble often stems from some hidden disease.

For *cardiac neurosis* see Chapter 12.

For *gastro-intestinal neurosis* see Chapter 13.

CHAPTER 12

DISORDERS OF THE HEART, CIRCULATION AND BLOOD VESSELS

The heart, circulation and blood vessels respond especially well to water treatments. The whole vascular system is toned up by them and reacts more as it should to external stimuli. There are also individual applications which have a special effect on the heart, while others act on the blood pressure. In every case, the water treatment must be supported by the appropriate diet and the exercises recommended by the doctor to suit the individual patient.

Abnormal Blood Pressure (Dysarteriotony)
People suffering from hypotonia, that is to say people whose blood pressure is too low, usually with a slower pulse rate than normal, suffer from disagreeable symptoms it is true but, because their whole heart and circulatory system is spared considerable stress, their life expectancy is higher than average. If the doctor finds nothing organically wrong that would call for treatment, the symptoms can be favourably influenced by gymnastics, exercising in the open air, air baths, cold affu-

sions, dew and water treading and contrast baths. In addition, garlic, mistletoe and hawthorn are given and, in certain circumstances a little champagne or coffee too (ask the doctor). It is typical of low blood pressure that the symptoms are better when the patient is lying down but are clearly aggravated when he stands up.

By way of contrast, high blood pressure must be always energetically treated. Constant medical supervision is necessary, for only the trained eye will recognize the possible secondary diseases in good time. A low salt diet is a prime element in any therapy, which will often be concerned with reducing weight as well. Harmful stimulants should be avoided and nicotine, as a vessel poison, is strictly forbidden. Regular exercise and breathing gymnastics, the absence of prolonged exertion of a physical or mental kind and a sensible attitude to life have as much to contribute to the reduction of the blood pressure as have arm baths and affusions, contrast foot baths, hip baths, relaxing hot complete baths or loin baths. Internally, garlic, mistletoe, hawthorn and onions are given. In special cases, the doctor will order rauwolfia preparations and other medicaments.

Arteriosclerotic changes in the blood vessels are irreversible. Hence prophyllaxis is vitally important. It is necessary to avoid prolonged stress, the abuse of nicotine and a diet that is too rich in fats and carbohydrates. High blood pressure and diabetes must receive treatment if present. High blood pressure and diabetes must receive treatment if present. In addition to this reformed diet and way of life, exercise in the open air is of great value.

In the place of animal fats, free use should be made of plant fats and oils containing unsaturated fatty acids, since these counteract the disease process. For internal use, garlic, mistletoe, hawthorn and the horsetail plant (rich in silicic acid) are to be recommended. As far as hydrotherapy is concerned, complete washes, knee and leg affusions and arm and foot baths may prove beneficial. When the sclerosis involves the cerebral blood vessels, tranquillizing herbs are often helpful, including, valerian, hops and St John's Wort oil. Permanent medical check-ups are necessary.

Cardiac Insufficiency (Heart Weakness)
Digitalis preparations as ordered by the doctor will form an important part of any therapy; in less serious cases hawthorn may also be employed. A low salt diet is absolutely necessary. In addition, breathing exercises (consult the doctor), cold washing of parts of the body, water treading, arm baths, arm and leg affusions are recommended.

Cardiac Neurosis
The first thing for the doctor to do in cardiac neurosis is to exclude the possibility of organic causes such as hormonal imbalance in puberty and at the change of life, disorders of the endocrine glands and deficiency diseases. In addition to the unpleasant heart symptoms there are usually other nervous symptoms as well.

Suitable preventive measures are breathing exercises, autogenic training, adequate exercise in the open air whatever the weather, valerian, hawthorn and strengthening baths and affusions. In some cases psychotherapy will be required. Cold heart compresses and graduated arm baths are good in acute cases. It is typical of the patient with cardiac neurosis to be very restless, whereas the person with an organic heart disease carefully spares his energies. Only the specialist can make a differential diagnosis, however.

Extrasystoles or heartbeats out of their proper order, frequently accompany a nervous disorder; but here again, only the doctor can ascertain the cause and order the proper treatment. Nervous extrasystoles, is treated by taking tranquillizing herbal teas, baths with valerian or rosemary added and using the above-mentioned packs, compresses or affusions.

Autogenic training also gives good results here.

Angina Pectoris
Attacks with an organic basis occur mostly in patients with high blood pressure, obesity or arteriosclerosis. Nearly all those affected are smokers. Similar troubles can arise from causes such as prolonged stress, general nerviness, the abuse of other stimulants, because the blood vessels

become cramped. However, attacks of angina pectoris can also be symptomatic of cardiac infarct and a medical examination is essential whenever they occur. The first step to take is to alter the life-style and to reduce mental tensions and conflicts. As in arteriosclerosis the food should contain vegetable fats and oils (unsaturated fatty acids) rather than animal fats. Alcoholic drinks and stimulants should be strictly avoided.

The therapy is supplemented, on the doctor's advice, by exercise in the open air, by graduated arm baths, arm and knee affusions and contrast foot baths.

Haemorrhoids (Piles)

Haemorrhoids announce themselves with itching of the anus, red stains or actual bleeding and even constipation as a reaction to the pain experienced when the bowels are evacuated. Frequent haemorrhages can lead to anaemia. The doctor should always be consulted, for some serious disease often lies behind the symptom of piles. Usually there is a constitutional weakness of the connective tissues which has been aggravated by obesity, chronic constipation, a sedentary life without much exercise, the abuse of alcohol and pregnancy. Part of the treatment is to keep the food soft by adoption of the proper diet. Plenty of exercise is also important. Special measures that can be taken are hip baths with oak-bark and camomile, vapour baths with the addition of camomile, and knee and leg affusions. Care must be taken that the anal region is kept clean after each evacuation (camomile, disinfectant solution). Tisanes made of stinging-nettle, camomile, yarrow, juniper and wormwood are taken internally, and local applications of horse-chestnut or pilewort ointment have also proved to be helpful, as have various medicated suppositories.

Varicose Veins

These changes in the condition of the veins are due partly to an inherited weakness of the connective tissue. Other causes are obesity, chronic constipation, frequently standing still, a lack of exercise and pregnancy. All these causes must be eliminated as far as possible. The best mode of prevention is to keep the foot of the bed permanently raised by about 30cm (1 foot). This measure is also useful as part of the basic treatment. The therapy should be supported by leg exercises, knee and leg affusions, contrast foot baths and water treading. Ointments applied locally usually contain horse chestnut and comfrey.

Crêpe bandages and rubber stockings are passive measures which give comfort but, in general, they should only be worn temporarily if the doctor approves. Medical check-ups are always necessary, since varicose veins can soon give rise to inflammation, thrombosis and finally embolism.

CHAPTER 13

DIGESTIVE AND METABOLIC DISTURBANCES

The wrong type of food, eaten in a rush in a mechanical way, and, in short, all the errors already pointed out in our chapter on a 'Well-balanced Diet', contribute to the digestive disorders that plague so many people today. Metabolic disturbances, too, especially diabetes, gout and obesity are also on the march.

The mental pressures on the person affected also play their part.

Gastro-intestinal Neurosis
A disagreeable sensation of pressure, cramps and colics in the region of the stomach and abdomen are often signs of a nervous dysfunction of the digestive organs. However, they may also be attributable to inflammations, ulcers and other organic diseases. When they continue for more than three days, the doctor must always be consulted.

In treating nervous disorders of the digestive system all the measures are basically indicated that are mentioned in the section on 'Nervousness'. Acute stomach ache is treated with camomile and balm tea and hot applications. Pressure on the stomach can be eased with gentian, wormwood, camomile tea and a short fast (one or two days). Cramps are usually quickly cured with hot compresses and packs, with camomile and balm tea and with deep breathing. If gastrectasia or gastroptosis (dilation of the stomach and downward displacement of the stomach respectively) are found to be the cause, water treading, washing the upper body, half baths, vinegar-water compresses are indicated for firming up the tissues.

Gastromucous Inflammation/Peptic ulcer

Acute inflammations of the mucous membrane of the stomach usually quickly abate, when one drinks nothing but unsugared camomile, peppermint or yarrow tea for two days.

Chronic inflammations require expert medical attention. The doctor should be given the opportunity of pointing out errors in the way of life and in the feeding habits. Hot packs half an hour before and after meals stimulate the stomach glands. Digestion is promoted by bitter herbs such as wormwood, calamus, centaury or gentian. Pineapple or patent enzyme preparations can substitute for missing enzymes. Tobacco and strong condiments must be strictly avoided. Autogenic training can deal with the mental causes.

The same applies to peptic and duodenal ulcers, in which worries always play a rôle. All the measures already described as beneficial in chronic gastritis are suitable for these ulcers. With the doctor's permission, cold body compresses can also be used for bleeding ulcers. Another possible form of treatment is where the patient drinks camomile or mallow tea or some solution prescribed by the doctor and then lies for five minutes on his back, right side, face and then left side. The cabbage or potato juice treatment (from health food stores) has proved to be exceptionally beneficial (duration 3 weeks). Liquorice juice is especially good in chronic ulcers, but, in view of the possibility of side-effects, it should be taken only under medical supervision.

Today the diet is no longer as stringent as it used to be a few years ago. What is important is that the food should be non-irritant, easily digestible, low-fat, not liable to cause flatulence and not too sweet. The daily intake of food is spread over 5 to 7 meals and thorough mastication is very important. Bicarbonate of soda should not be taken for heart-burn, because a build-up of gas in the stomach might cause a perforation of the ulcer if the worst came to the worst.

Gastro-enteritis/Diarrhoea

Inflammation of the mucous membranes is quite common. Self-treatment is permissible only in simple cases where there is no impairment of the general condition. As long as the diarrhoea persists, only camomile and peppermint tea are taken. Later the patient starts on a diet of apple and unsweetened whortleberries (bilberries) and then gradually returns to his usual full diet. The hydrotherapeutic treatments indicated include hot hay-seed and steam compresses on the abdomen, complete baths with hayseed, washing of the upper body, vinegar-water washes and hot foot baths.

Especially in short attacks of diarrhoea, astringent teas such as oak bark and tormentil, and in addition camomile, sage, centaury, wormwood or whortleberry (bilberry) juice, are helpful.

Constipation

Chronic constipation is one of the scourges of modern civilization and is particularly common among women. The regular use of laxatives is always harmful. Training the bowels to be punctual is of fundamental importance, and so is the inclusion of a certain amount of roughage in the food. And the visit should not be too brief.

Constipation can usually be overcome by eating wholemeal and linseed bread, a few figs in the morning or prunes that have been soaked in water, taken on an empty stomach. In stubborn cases, an aperient herbal tea or garlic or rhubarb juice will generally provoke a motion. If none of these measures work then it is time to call in the doctor.

Flatulence

Attacks of flatulence have very various causes and can be a pointer to serious organic diseases. However, they are often due to nervous air-swallowing. Only the doctor can make a definite diagnosis.

When the causes are nervous, the same means are used as are mentioned under 'Nervousness'. Generally speaking, fennel, caraway seed, peppermint and hot body packs with vinegar-water are indicated and, in addition, complete washing, leg affusions and contrast hip baths.

Obesity

Prominent in the treatment is some form of diet, as ordered by the doctor. This will be rich in low-calorie uncooked food without cooking salt or animal fat.

Gymnastics and plenty of exercise in the open air are indicated for regulating the metabolism. Supportive measures are the short compress, the Spanish Cloak, hot complete baths, various affusions, and teas made with bladderwrack, watercress, fumitory, black alder bark and other vegetable remedies.

Gout

Although there is doubtless a certain hereditary pre-disposition to gout, this disease is mainly brought about by rich feeding. The things to avoid are alcohol, dark meat that is rich in uric acid, chocolate and other foodstuffs with a high uric acid content. A meatless diet may be advised by the practitioner also. The measures to be adopted for acute involvement of the joints are hot complete baths with the addition of oatstraw or hayseed, hot oatstraw, potato and hayseed sacks, full steam baths, hayseed shirts and hayseed contrast foot baths. Later, cold complete washes, affusions, half baths, Spanish Cloaks and water treading are indicated. Constant medical supervision is always indicated because of the threat of secondary diseases.

Diabetes

The diet of someone suffering from diabetes will always be decided by the therapist and it would exceed the limits of this book to discuss it in detail here. Nevertheless, the proper diet is of crucial importance for holding the disease permanently in check.

Hydrotherapy recommends morning complete washes, short compresses, leg and upper body affusions and Spanish Cloaks, and afternoon applications of arm baths, knee affusions, arm affusions, body packs and hayseed sacks on the epigastrium. In addition, it is necessary for the diabetic to take plenty of exercise in the open air and to perform regular gymnastic exercises. Oatmeal days and various medicinal herbs are often all that is needed with a natural diabetic diet but, in serious cases, the patient will not be able to do without insulin. This will be prescribed by the doctor in charge when necessary and the latter will also keep the general condition of the patient under constant review.

CHAPTER 14

DISEASES OF THE BONES AND JOINTS AND OTHER DISORDERS

The patients whom the general practitioner sees in his surgery will be suffering from one or other of these diseases more often than not. Scarcely a single human being goes through life without some personal experience of them. Now, in many cases, excellent results are obtained in treating disorders of the bones and joints by using the Kneipp applications either, as the sole form of treatment or else as supportive therapy.

Arthritis/Arthropathy
Whenever inflammation of the joints is present, the doctor should be called in to prevent destruction of the articular cartilage and the onset of chronic arthrosis.

The internal treatment consists of willowbark tea; externally the affected joints are washed with vinegar-water and affusions and, as healing progresses, massage and exercise in the open air are indicated.

In arthropathy which is a chronic degenerative disease and irreversible, and more usual in elderly patients, sting-ing nettle, dandelion and juniper-berry tea are given internally. The affected joints are treated locally with mud-baths, hot hayseed sacks and sweating cures.

Lumbago/Backache

Quite often, backache is the symptom of some other trouble with the pain referred to the lumbar region from elsewhere. In women, especially, abdominal trouble must always be considered. When the doctor has ruled out such organic causes, recourse may be made to arnica and salicylic acid ointments, vapour baths, hot hayseed sacks and massage.

Backache is usually the symptom of disc trouble and will require the doctor's attention. Local applications which have proved their value are hayseed sacks, hot packs, steam compresses, vinegar-water washes and, at a later stage, short compresses, loin and back affusions, graduated hayseed baths and hot complete or half baths. In addition, ointments containing arnica or St John's Wort and peppermint oil can soothe the pain. Birch and willow teas, taken internally, are also beneficial.

Sciatica

This very painful process sometimes arises from disc trouble, but can also be caused by inflammations, lesions and metabolic disorders. For this reason, it is essential to take professional advice. The pain shoots right down to the foot. Sometimes the services of an osteopath or chiropractor are indicated.

The basic therapy consists of steam compresses, hot packs, cold compresses round the calves and hot foot baths, with later, contrast foot baths and contrast hip baths, leg affusions and hot complete baths. St John's Wort oil, peppermint oil and lavender oil make a good embrocation and herbal teas for rheumatism can be taken internally.

Rheumatism

Rheumatism occurs in a number of different forms. Sometimes it is acute, sometimes chronic; at times it attacks the joints and at times it also attacks the soft parts of the body. Because there is a threat of secondary diseases and the possibility of disablement, rheumatism is a serious disease that requires professional treatment.

Exceptionally good results have often been obtained by thrashing the skin with stinging nettles and by drinking stinging nettle, dandelion and juniper berry tea. Local applications consist of affusions, hayseed compresses, clay and vinegar-water packs and ointments containing arnica, comfrey, menthol, peppermint, rosemary and other herbal remedies. For muscular rheumatism hot hayseed baths, cold affusions and washes in vinegar-water are indicated, while poplar and willow bark tea are taken internally. Whipping the affected part with stinging nettle leaves has often been beneficial too.

Each form of rheumatism must be properly cleared up and, when this has been done, a complete medical check-up will be required to ensure that there are no after-effects or permanent damage.

As has been said, the Kneipp system is suitable for the prevention and treatment of practically all diseases. Therefore, what we say here must, of necessity, be very incomplete and limited to the most important disorders. But here are a few more troubles for which the Kneipp treatments will be found useful.

Menstrual Disorders and The Change of Life

It goes without saying that the doctor must be consulted where menstrual disorders are concerned. Kneipp treatments should only be attempted with such approval. Exercise in the open air and correction of the frequently present constipation are always in order. Good results have been obtained by hot abdominal packs, cold hip baths, contrast hip baths and half baths, wet socks, loin compresses, foot baths and cold head compresses. Herbal teas to be taken include shepherd's purse, ragwort, horsetail and lady's mantle. The psychological condition of the woman must also be considered.

The troubles associated with the change of life, which generally pass fairly quickly where there has been adequate preparation for and adjustment to this new phase of life, can (with medical permission) be treated by means of baths containing valerian, by hip baths and contrast baths with horsetail plant, contrast foot baths, graduated arm baths, complete washes and various forms of affusion. Among the herbs used internally, lady's mantle, shepherd's purse, St John's Wort, rosemary and common yarrow are recommended. The food should be non-stimulating. Regular medical check-ups are especially important during the menopause.

Heat-stroke/Sunstroke

Heat-stroke is the consequence of reduced perspiration that leads to caloric stasis in the body. Suitable clothing can usually be relied on to prevent this trouble. As soon as heat-stroke is suspected, with the sufferer possibly having lost consciousness, the latter individual is immediately removed to a shady spot and his upper body is sprinkled with cold water, which is quickly evaporated by fanning him with a cloth.

Further treatment may be given with packs laid on the head, chest and abdomen, if the doctor permits, or by cold foot baths.

Sunstroke, due to direct exposure of the uncovered head to the sun, can occur 12 hours later. It must always be treated by the doctor. As an emergency measure, treat as for heat-stroke. To draw the trouble away from the head, use arm baths, compresses on the arms, legs, calves, feet and loins, and try water treading and wet socks. Strong coffee can be administered if the patient is conscious. To be on the safe side, one should never go out in the hot sun without having the head covered.

Fever

Fever is to be treated only when it has lasted too long or the temperature is too high since, in most cases, it is a useful defence mechanism.

Complete washing with vinegar-water, calf compresses, and decoctions of willow bark are usually permitted and, when there are chills, an initial graduated half bath followed by a two-hour dry-pack with hot water bottles, with elder and lime-flower tea to drink, and finally a cold wash. The doctor must always be called in when the fever lasts for any length of time or if one is uncertain about its nature.

Cold in the Head

Inhalations with camomile tea to which a few drops of eucalyptus oil or thyme oil have been added have proved to be especially efficacious for relieving colds. Nasal irrigation with lemon juice, camomile or horsetail herb tea or cooking salt solution is also indicated. An old domestic remedy was snuffing iodine up the nose, but this is injurious and most definitely must not be used.

In chronic nasal catarrh, dispersive treatments such as leg affusions, complete washes with vinegar water and half baths are indicated. Ointments containing marjoram or origanum (wild marjoram) are also helpful.

Hay Fever

Hay fever is given dispersive treatment away from the head with water treading, half baths, hot complete baths, leg affusions, and nasal irrigation as mentioned above plus teas of eyebright, pimpernel, lungwort, marigold and wormwood. If possible, desensitizing should be carried out, but this is a matter for the doctor to decide. The best thing for inflammation of the nasal sinuses is to breathe camomile vapour with the addition of thyme oil. Externally, fenugreek and hayseed packs are applied, together with dispersive treatments such as leg and upperbody affusions and short compresses. In all illnesses involving the nose, a low-liquid diet is important.

Frigidity/Impotence

These two forms of sexual disorder are nearly always psychological in origin and often require psychotherapy. A cure is almost always possible, and the doctor should be consulted in each case. Kneipp treatments can effectively support the main therapy.

In frigidity, most benefit has been obtained from graduated hip baths and hot jets of water on the lumbar area of the spine. In impotence, pelvic affusions have proved helpful together with tranquillizing herbs which will reduce anxiety over failure on the part of the man.

CHAPTER 15

HOME AIDS TO HEALTH

Back-brush
The brush should be made with natural bristles and should not be too hard. It is essential for it to have a handle that is at least 40cm (16 ins) long so that there is no difficulty in reaching any part of the body. The latest brushes have hollow handles into which a shower-rose or bubble-bath attachment can be screwed. The brush is used for soaping and the skin is massaged at the same time.

Sponge
A hard natural sponge can replace the back-brush, but it is more difficult to reach certain parts of the body with it. The sponge also enables the person taking a bath to massage and soap themselves at the same time.

Massage Glove
The rough bath glove made of friction cloth is used for massaging the body when soaping or drying it. As in the case of the sponge, it is not easy to reach all parts of the body with it.

Back Massager
This has been devised especially for massaging the back.

The back massager consists of a wide band of rough material with two handles and is easily drawn over the back.

The brush, sponge, glove and back massager are employed either for dry massage or during and after the bath. Daily massage stimulates the skin and improves its circulation.

Bath Tubs
The shape and size of the bath tub will depend on the type of bath being taken. Even washtubs or pails will serve for foot baths. Arm baths can be carried out in the wash-basin. Special tubs for hip baths can be purchased from the ironmonger. However, it is only worthwhile buying one when hip baths are taken frequently, otherwise any other suitable tub will do in which one can sit with the water coming up to the kidneys and covering the thighs. Half baths and hip baths are taken in the ordinary domestic bath tub but the latter will generally be too short for complete baths up to the neck. It is better to do without a complete bath rather than to double up awkwardly in a tub that is really too small.

Foot Rollers
This consists of two 'wheels' joined by a corrugated cylinder. It is placed under the feet and moved backwards and forwards in such a way that the soles of the feet from the heels to the toes are well massaged. The effect can be felt in the calf muscles.

Hot Water Bottles
These are required for soothing local discomfort of the type that responds to warmth, for example rheumatic pain, and for conserving the heat in hot compresses.

Artificial Sunlight/Solarium
When days are dark and cold, artificial sunlight or a solarium can substitute for the summer sun. Good sun-lamps are fitted with a safety-switch, a timer alarm, filters and skin-type selector. They radiate ultra-violet light within a limited range together with infra-red light. The lamp is usually set three feet (1 metre, approx.) away from

the body and the length of each exposure is adjusted according to the sensitivity of the patient and the maker's instructions. Where there is any doubt, a start should be made with the shortest exposure time. A solarium irradiates the whole body and must be fitted with a two-phase switch for radiation at ordinary strength when the filters are open and at greater intensity when the filters are closed; in this way the skin will be protected from an overdose. Good models are also equipped with signals that warn when the filters are open, with a time-switch, distance measurer, and protective screen and work with a combination of ultra-violet and infra-red radiation. Sometimes they are permanently fixed to the wall or ceiling and sometimes they are mounted on a mobile support. The excessive use of either type is injurious to health and in certain circumstances can increase the risk of skin cancer.

Massage Douche

This differs from the usual rose belonging to the bathroom shower because of the special arrangement of the spray-holes. By massage with fine jets of water, the skin is toned up, the muscles are relaxed and the circulation is improved. The new rose can be substituted for the old in a matter of minutes.

There is a special type of massage douche for imparting a good shape to the female bust. It fits like a cup over the breast and the water spurts from the small holes under fairly high pressure, so that the whole surface circulation of the breast is stimulated, the skin is toned up and excess fat is reduced.

Infra-red Lamps

Long-wave radiation from the infra-red end of the spectrum is suitable for alleviating pain and for many forms of inflammation. Preferably, the doctor will be consulted before using it, since at a certain stage in head colds the heat can change simple catarrh to a blockage of the nasal sinuses. In good sun-lamps, the ultra-violet radiation can be switched off so that the infra-red light may be used on its own.

Vibrators
Vibration massage using light, continuous vibrations improves the circulation of the blood and reduces local accumulations of fat. The vibrator is a piece of massage equipment in which an alternating current with a frequency of 50 cycles per second imparts the finest vibrations to an iron core. This equipment has proved helpful in the relief of mild headaches. There are special vibrator cups for toning up the female breast too.

Exercise Cycle
These home trainers will help all those who have little time to spend on keeping fit. They have a lever for adjusting the resistance of the pedals, so that the effect can be increased without taking any more time. Where there is a tendency to varicose veins, the home trainer must not be used unless the doctor allows it. The rowing-machine exercises more muscles than the exercise cycle does. Here too the effort can be adjusted as required.

INDEX

Angina pectoris, 79-80
Affusions, 35-43
Anxiety, 75
Arm affusion, 36-7
  bath, 48
  compresses, 24, 25
Arthritis, 87-8
Arthropathy, 87-8

Backache, 88
Back affusion, 39-40
  packs, 32
Bath additives, 46-7
Baths, 46-8, 51
  sun and air, 64
Blood pressure (abnormal), 77-8
Body packs, 32
Breathing exercises, 62-3

Calf compresses, 25
Cardiac insufficiency, 79
Cardiac neurosis, 79
Cataplasms, 34
Change of life, 89-90
Chest compress, 26
Chest-to-toe compress, 28
Compresses, 22-34
  cold, 23
  cross-over, 27
  full, 29-30
  hot, 23
  short, 28
  slap-on, 34
Constipation, 84
Curds, in compress, 32

Depression, 75
Diabetes, 85-6
Diarrhoea, 84
Diet, 11-12, 66-71
Dispersion, 59
Dysarteriotony, 77

Equipment, for treatment, 92-5
Exercise, 60-62
Eye bath, 50

Face affusion, 39
  bath, 50
Fever, 23, 90
Flatulence, 84-5
Fomentations, 33
Foot bath, 49, 50
Foot compresses, 25
Frigidity, 91
Front packs, 32

Gastro-enteritis, 84
Gastro-intestinal neurosis, 82-3
Gastromucous inflammation, 83
Gout, 85

Haemorrhoids, 80

Half bath, 51
Half vapour bath, 56-7
Hand compress, 24-5
Hay fever, 91
Headache, 75
Head affusion, 39
  cold, 91
  compress, 25-6
Healing crisis, 15-16
Heart weakness, 79
Heat stroke, 90
Hip bath, 50
Holistic therapy, 9
Hot rollers, 34
How You Should Live, 17

Impotence, 91

Jets, 43-5

Knee affusion, 37-8
  jet, 43

Leg affusion, 38
  jet, 43

Loin compress, 28
Lower body affusion, 41
Lower-leg bath, 49
  compress, 25
Lumbago, 88

Menstrual disorders, 89
Migraine, 75-6

Neck compress, 26
Nervousness, 74

Obesity, 85
Open-air baths, 64

Peptic ulcers, 83-4
Piles, 80

Rheumatism, 88-9

Sacks, 34
Sauna, 53
Sciatica, 88
Shawl treatment, 31-2
Shirt treatment, 30
Sleep disorders, 74-5
Spanish cloak treatment, 30
Steam bath, 53
Sun baths, 64-5
Sun stroke, 90

Upper body affusion, 39

Vapour baths, 53, 54, 57-8
Vapour treatment, 52-9
Varicose veins, 80-81

Washing, 20-21
Water treading, 58-9
Wet sock treatment, 32
Whole leg compress, 25